# Community College Student Mental Health

# THE FUTURES SERIES ON COMMUNITY COLLEGES

Richard L. Alfred, series founding editor, Emeritus Professor of Higher Education, University of Michigan; Debbie L. Sydow, series senior editor, president, Richard Bland College of the College of William and Mary; and Kate Thirolf, series editor, associate professor, Community College Policy and Administration, University of Maryland Global Campus.

*The Futures Series on Community Colleges* is designed to produce and deliver books that strike to the heart of issues that will shape the future of community colleges. *Futures* books examine emerging structures, systems and business models, and stretch prevailing assumptions about leadership and management by reaching beyond the limits of convention and tradition.

## Books in Series

# Community College Student Mental Health

## Faculty Experiences and Institutional Actions

Amanda O. Latz

ROWMAN & LITTLEFIELD
Lanham • Boulder • New York • London

Published by Rowman & Littlefield
An imprint of The Rowman & Littlefield Publishing Group, Inc.
4501 Forbes Boulevard, Suite 200, Lanham, Maryland 20706
www.rowman.com

86-90 Paul Street, London EC2A 4NE, United Kingdom

British Library Cataloguing in Publication Information Available

**Library of Congress Cataloging-in-Publication Data**

Names: Latz, Amanda O., author.
Title: Community college student mental health : faculty experiences and institutional
    actions / Amanda O. Latz.
Description: Lanham, Maryland : Rowman & Littlefield, 2023. | Series: The futures
    series on community colleges | Includes bibliographical references. | Summary: "This
    book is focused on community college student mental health, which is a critical topic
    among community college leaders, faculty, and staff"—Provided by publisher.
Identifiers: LCCN 2023017192 (print) | LCCN 2023017193 (ebook) | ISBN
    9781475860153 (cloth) | ISBN 9781475860160 (paperback) | ISBN
    9781475860177 (epub)
Subjects: LCSH: Counseling in higher education—United States. | Community college
    students—Mental health—United States. | Community college students—Mental
    health services—United States.
Classification: LCC LB2343 .L328 2023  (print) | LCC LB2343  (ebook) | DDC
    378.1/9713—dc23/eng/20230418
LC record available at https://lccn.loc.gov/2023017192
LC ebook record available at https://lccn.loc.gov/2023017193

♾™ The paper used in this publication meets the minimum requirements of American
National Standard for Information Sciences—Permanence of Paper for Printed Library
Materials, ANSI/NISO Z39.48-1992.

*This book is dedicated to the faculty who shared their stories with me. It was my honor and pleasure to be in your presence, have important conversations, and feel alongside each and all of you.*

# Contents

# Acknowledgments

It has taken me a long time to write this book. Many, many people helped me along the way. I would like to first thank my family. My partner of nearly 21 years, Annette, has been a constant supporter and source of inspiration. Her gentle directives like, "Go write your book," were always meant lovingly and helped me make space for the necessary work—even when it was really, really hard. Thank you, and I love you. My parents never tired of me talking about how "I have got to get this book done." I appreciate and love you both very much. My menagerie of pets over the past few years have also played a part in making this book happen, especially during the pandemic. To my critters past and present, Scooter, Wink, Muncie, Red, Yellow, Slick, Backpack, Lemon, Fizz, The Mollies, Snizz, Fluff, and Dottie, I love you all so much. Thank you for understanding when I was paying so much attention to my laptop. Thank you for lending a paw, wing, fin, and foot when I needed you. Several thought partners and readers coached me through early chapter drafts. To Jeffry Neuhouser, Carrie Rodesiler, Sam Snideman, Ashleigh Bingham, who are current and former students, I so appreciate all your thoughtful and useful feedback. I am especially thankful for Jeffry Neuhouser, who knows me well enough to comment on whether pieces of writing sound like me or not—and helping me hone *my* voice through writing. To Karen Hansen-Morgan, thank you for the exquisite editing support. I would also like to thank the many colleagues and students who have heard me talk about this book over the years. And, finally, to Kate Thirolf, I had no idea how important and awesome our author-editor relationship would be until we got into the thick of revisions. Wow. Innumerable thanks for all the time and attention you gave to my writing. You enhanced this manuscript in so many ways. Because of you, the book is well-organized, easy to read, and accessible to a broad audience. Thank you also for believing in this book and knowing how much it is needed right now.

I also want to thank readers. While it feels good to have written this book, and while I am very proud of it, I did not do this work for me. I did this work for community college students. And I did this work for community college faculty. You, dear reader, picked up this book for a reason. Now it is time for you to do the work.

# Chapter 1

# Introduction

"This is such a great study. When I saw it, I said, 'This is perfect.'"

—Camille

Though not always noticeable, many community college students have diagnosed mental illness(es) or experience symptoms that suggest the existence of a mental health issue or concern. Student mental health is a profound issue facing all of higher education, and it is most pronounced within the community college sector. There is no evidence to suggest this issue is going to become less pronounced; in fact, the opposite is the case.

While the literature on this topic has grown by leaps and bounds since 2015, it remains underdeveloped. This book is meant to provide three things: (a) an overview of what is already known on the topic; (b) a detailed explanation of a study I carried out on the topic; and (c) a set of institutional actions that can be implemented by institutional agents to address, and, at least partially, redress the issue.

During the spring semester of 2017, I interviewed 22 community college faculty about their students' mental health. At the time, I was not able to locate any literature on community college faculty experiences with or perceptions of their students' mental health, and Brenda Kucirka noted the same gap within the four-year institution context.[1] While a gap in the literature does not automatically mean it should be filled, I knew faculty insights on this topic would be invaluable to understanding it.

This was more than a research study for me. Through the entirety of the experience, I came into solidarity with these astutely committed educators who work tirelessly each day to create meaningful and effective learning environments for students. As a former community college faculty member myself,[2] our interviews became more like conversations between trusted friends.

1

The talk was emotive, empathic, and important. There was trust, vulnerability, and bravery. There is much to share from these exchanges that might assist a broad audience in thinking not only about community college student mental health, but also the lives of community college faculty.

Community college faculty are critical to the success of community college students. The community college student experience—and community college student success—is largely characterized by academic tethers to the institution.[3] These tethers include, for example, academic integration,[4] academic validation,[5] socio-academic integrative moments,[6] and contact with faculty,[7] both inside and outside of the institution. Social tethers such as peer connections and involvement with institutional organizations seem to play less of a role in student success within the community college as compared to the four-year sector.

Community college faculty are vital components of students' academic tethers to their institution. Therefore, community college faculty are vital to community college students. My lived experiences, research activities in this area, and review of the extant literature point to the centrality of faculty-student interactions, connections, and relationships throughout community colleges across the United States. Understanding community college students through the lenses of their faculty has efficacy heretofore not fully realized. My aim is to redress that under-realization through this book—at least in part.

Community college student mental health has recently become a critical issue, which has been exacerbated by the COVID-19 pandemic. Yet very few studies exist related to the mental health of community college students.[8] *At least* 50 percent of community college students—one of every two—is currently living with a mental health issue of some kind, and only half of those students are receiving services.[9]

These issues include anxiety, depression, post-traumatic stress, bipolar disorder, and schizophrenia, just to name a few broad categories of examples. Living with and managing poor mental health may include cultivating coping strategies, accessing and affording care, accessing and affording prescription medication, and negotiating the myriad stigmas associated with mental health. As compared with their counterparts at four-year institutions, community college students have more mental health issues and fewer institutional resources,[10] making this a substantial concern for community college campus agents.[11]

Supporting students' mental health within the community college sector is no easy or simple task. In 2015, Alan Schwitzer and Brian Van Brunt noted that community colleges face unique challenges in supporting students with mental health disorders on campus.[12] One factor is the additional duties many on-campus mental health counselors must carry out as a part of their responsibilities, which, in some cases, includes academic support services such as advising. This is corroborated by much of the literature outlined in chapter 3.

Many community college students arrive on campus with a higher likelihood for attrition than their counterparts at four-year institutions, and when considering that community college students are more likely to have mental health problems, "the stress and potential for an acute crisis rise considerably . . . [and] staff can become frustrated and overwhelmed in the face of enormous need and limited resources."[13]

While the literature on this topic is proliferating, most extant studies have been approached quantitatively and centered on the students themselves, rather than community college campus agents' understandings of students' mental health. However, grasping the ways *faculty* understand community college students' mental health can provide unique insights related to the core issue at hand: effectively supporting community college students through their educational journeys toward completion. Furthermore, Paula E. McBride called for studies that "indicate how students and/or staff or *faculty* perceive the need for mental health services on a two-year campus."[14] She called for a study like this.

Because most community colleges are commuter institutions, with students often only accessing campus for class attendance, faculty tend to have the most contact with students, as compared to other campus agents, such as academic advisors, residence hall personnel, or librarians. To many community college students, their faculty *are* their community college,[15] and engagement with faculty, both inside and outside the classroom, can have significant impacts on students' success.[16]

As such, understanding faculty perceptions can provide a more holistic view of this topic, giving way to nuanced and potentially more effective pedagogies, support strategies, policies, and infrastructure to scaffold students as they pursue their postsecondary educational goals. Alan M. "Woody" Schwitzer and John A. Vaughn said they "know that professionals from every corner of campus can describe first-hand how students' mental and physical wellness, or lack thereof, can affect their learning and success,"[17] yet the current literature base is lacking in empirical evidence to support this claim.

The purpose of my study was to shed light on how community college faculty understand their students' mental health. Community college faculty can and do play a role in supporting students living with a mental health concern. Considering the primacy of faculty in community college students' lives and the prevalence of this issue, understanding what faculty have to say about it is critical.[18] This perspective is largely absent in the literature, yet we cannot afford this inattention any longer.

Many faculty are well aware that some students in their classrooms are likely managing symptoms of poor mental health such as tiredness, inability to focus, mood swings, or even physical pain. The conversations I had with these faculty members were rich with stories, suggestions, and perspectives from individuals who regularly interact with students on an intimate level. Within this book, I amplify their voices on this issue and make suggestions regarding what the future landscape might look like with regards to community college student mental health and the faculty who support these students.

Within qualitative research, researcher reflexivity is paramount. This is especially the case with reflexive thematic analysis,[19] which I used for this book. As such, who I am as a researcher and interpreter of data ought to be shared with the work's audiences as a means of bolstering trustworthiness.[20]

It is incumbent upon qualitative researchers, then, to share aspects of their personhoods and positionality relative to the focus of any given topic(s) of study. To share some insights into who I am, included below is a relevant vignette, or personal narrative. I wrote this piece well over 10 years ago as the beginning pages of my doctoral dissertation and deliberated on whether to include it here. In the end, I decided it is a story worth telling. This narrative will provide readers with views into my pedagogy and philosophy as a former community college faculty member—as well as some of the ways I have interacted with community college students throughout the years.

## AN AGED VIGNETTE

Only upon reflection am I able to realize that I was totally out of my element at the time. When experiencing flow, or a period of being completely absorbed in an activity, individuals have no room in their consciousness to think about themselves.[21] In other words, when in flow, self-consciousness disappears.

I was at a bar downtown known for hosting live music. I was belly up to a strip of caution tape that was being used to close off a rectangular area in the middle of the bar and in front of the stage, and I had been holding the same empty bottle of beer for almost three hours. It just never crossed my mind to go back to the bar for another drink. This was not a typical evening out for me. And much to my surprise, I was completely enthralled by the scene that unfolded in front of me. There was a lot of activity around me, but I was focused on the spectacle directly in my line of sight.

Let me provide some context. It was late January of 2009. The spring semester was in its beginning stages. I was teaching *Cultural Anthropology* and *First-Year Seminar* at a local community college. In the anthropology course, the capstone project was called the Exploration Project (in hindsight and with my current understanding about the problematic colonial history of the field of anthropology, I would change the name of this project). Students self-selected cultures to study and were encouraged to choose a culture that was personally meaningful.

The process of selecting a topic of study began on the first day of class. Through in-class discussions, email correspondence, and face-to-face communication, I helped students arrive at their topics. At the time, the Exploration Project included a written paper, an in-class presentation, and a public open house. Some students are hesitant to select sensitive or controversial topics for fear of offending others. This was especially the case for one of my students that semester. Recall that these projects are seen by me, their classmates, and whoever attends the open house. I will call my student Kevin (pseudonym).

On the very first day of class, I showed a documentary film titled *Metal: A Headbanger's Journey* made by an anthropologist and heavy metal fan, Sam Dunn, about the culture of heavy metal music: the bands, key figures, fans, concerts, history, clothing, symbols, world views, and values. Kevin was a metal fan and a bass player for a local metal band. After I showed the film, Kevin and I, unbeknownst to me at the time, had common ground. I was not a metal fan, but I was aware of it enough to show a film about it.

As such, Kevin felt at least some sense of comfort with me and soon approached me about his Exploration Project topic, and did so very early, within the first two weeks of the semester. When he first approached me, I could tell he was a bit tentative. He explained his idea but had basically rejected it before he even voiced it to me. He was concerned that the content would be too off-putting to his classmates and those who would attend the open house. He was interested in completing his project on the culture of suspension arts.

Kevin was a suspension artist and wanted to educate others on this frequently misunderstood culture. However, he had experienced a lot of negative feedback and disapproval about being a part of this culture from various individuals, especially within the educational context we were sharing. During our conversations about his idea, he shared with me that once, upon disclosing his involvement in suspension arts, one of his instructors insisted that he seek psychological counseling. This was an example of misunderstanding.

So, what is suspension art? In suspension arts, the body is pierced by large hooks in various places such as the back, chest, arms, belly, knees, or legs. Then, the hooks are connected, with rope, to a metal bracing. The bracing hangs from a pulley, which is connected to the ceiling or other high structure. Rock climbing rope is used to connect the bracing, through the pulley, to a person who is anchored to the ground and wearing a harness, much like a belay system.

The person anchored to the ground, or the belayer, hoists the person being suspended into the air with nothing keeping them (singular they) off the ground aside from the hooks in their flesh. Now it may be clearer why Kevin was apprehensive about his potential project topic and why, without understanding the culture, someone might assume a suspension artist needs psychological counseling.

It is important to note that in early January of 2009, I had only a foggy and ill-informed idea of what suspension art was. I recalled seeing something about it on television, but that was the extent of my knowledge. I was upfront with Kevin about this. I also made it quite clear I thought he should pursue the topic. I asked him about why he engaged in suspension, along with a myriad of other questions. I was interested in knowing why he did it, what it provided him, and how he got started.

Much to my surprise, Kevin had a hard time articulating answers to my questions. Most surprisingly, he could not articulate why he did it. He knew why he did it, but he could not explain it to me. I asked him where he suspended. This would prove to be a critical question. He responded by saying in the woods, in airplane hangars, at tattoo conventions, and in bars. Shows in bars were open to the public.

He casually mentioned that he had a show coming up in town. And almost as an afterthought, he said that I should come. At that moment, I began fighting the twinge of discomfort that began to form inside me. The acquisition of facts seemed to be the best defense. What would it be like? Who would be there? How would I fit in? His responses seemed satisfactory, and I told him that I would consider it.

By the time the next week arrived, Kevin's request for me to see his show had amplified. He had spoken to some of the others involved with the show and the consensus was that I should go to the show. In fact, Kevin said that one of the other people involved in the show said that I, as an instructor of *cultural* anthropology, *needed* to go.

Not being one to back down from a perceived challenge, I asked him for the details and told him I would be there. I thought intensely about going alone or trying to recruit friends to join me, what I would wear, if I would have a drink, what I would do if I became uncomfortable, when I would arrive and depart, and what it would be like to witness a suspension show.

I recruited two others to join me at the show; that was comforting. When we first arrived at the bar, I felt out of place. Nothing in particular made me feel out of place. It was simply my own self-consciousness and insecurity. All the other attendees seemed to be welcoming or otherwise indifferent to the three of us. While we did not completely blend into the crowd, we did not draw any attention either. Kevin greeted us gleefully and did not stop smiling until it was time for him to begin preparing for his suspension. When we arrived, there were not too many people at the bar, so we were able to get really close to the performance area.

Back to the opening paragraph of this vignette. After grabbing a Bud Light from the bar, the three of us stepped up to the caution tape that quarantined the suspension area. The tape was strung around a large metal rack. It reminded me of a squat rack seen inside gyms, but bigger, larger in width, length, and height. The rack consumed about a 12-foot by 12-foot area. We were standing at what I will call the front of the rack, and a stage, which would soon house a metal band, stood behind the rack.

In the suspensions area, there was plastic sheeting on the floor, a table that looked like it belonged in a medical facility, and plastic containers of sundry medical supplies like gauze, hermetically sealed instruments, ointments, and antiseptics. As I described above, the bracing rack was hanging from a pulley attached to the ceiling, and there was a harness splayed out on the floor.

People were bustling around, and the band was getting ready to start in the background. The first person to suspend was a younger man probably in his early twenties. He had a small to medium build and a few tattoos. The person who appeared to be in charge served the roles of medical technician, piercer, and belayer.

This person had blond dreaded hair, a large beard, lots of tattoos and facial piercings, large spacers in his ear lobes, and a look of intense focus in his eyes. This man, whom I will call the master of ceremonies, smoked a lot of cigarettes and was all business the entire time. His gaze rarely left the suspension area, and his eyes were constantly on those suspended in the air once they got there. It was his job to cut them down and to decide when the limits were being pushed too far.

We watched the first individual to be suspended undergo the preparation rituals: focusing the mind, drinking beer and smoking cigarettes, smiling at the growing crowd as his back and knees were doused with betadine, turning away as the hooks were pushed through his flesh, and jumping and bouncing around as he prepared to be attached to the bracing rack. As this was happening, Kevin paced around the bar with a nervous, yet excited, energy.

He checked in with us to chat several times as we watched his fellow suspension artists prepare. We had a lot of questions. The first individual was attached to the bracing rack by four hooks in his back, spaced out evenly. After the attachment, the master of ceremonies strung the climbing rope, which was strung through the pulley, through the carabiner, which was attached to his harness, and tied a beautifully intricate knot. Somehow, the master of ceremonies then braced himself and hoisted the suspender up into the air.

At this point, we all held our breath. There was no way of knowing what to expect. His flesh moved up before he did, and I was not sure how far it would go before his feet would leave the ground. He was giving the crowd a slightly crooked smile. He seemed like a little kid about to do something he knew he would get in trouble for later.

Once the suspended man was at the appropriate height, the master of ceremonies somehow secured the rope. The master of ceremonies no longer needed the harness to keep the suspended man in the air. Once in the air, the man seemed to have no pain. By this point, the band was playing, and it was almost as if he were dancing. Next, it was Kevin's turn to be pierced. I felt maternal and affected. I did not want to see my student in pain but came to realize later that he was never really in pain. Kevin had four hooks placed in his knees, two in each. We were not sure what would happen next.

With the hooks in, Kevin approached us and introduced us to his mom, who was also in the audience. She talked to us and reminded all of us to keep an open mind. That conversation was among one of the last things I expected to happen that night. After the last pre-suspension visit with Kevin, we learned that he was going to be connected to the man already suspended. Kevin's knees would be tied to the man's knees. They would both be held in the air by the hooks in the man's back.

Surprisingly, I was becoming more and more unaware of everything that was happening except for the act of suspension in front of me. Gradually, I was less and less concerned with myself and whether I was an appropriate fit in the scene. Kevin spent a brief period above the ground attached to the suspended man.

After this performance, Kevin carried out a solo suspension. After watching the suspensions intently for about three hours, the three of us decided to head home. As we drove away from the bar, we all reflected on the experience and how fascinating it was. It was nothing like we had expected it to be. There was no carnage, cries of pain, or difficult things to watch.

The next time I saw Kevin in class, he almost had a swagger and look on his face that suggested he felt that we had grown closer because of the suspension show. He told me that later in the evening the drummer of the band that was playing during the suspension show said to him, "Dude, my old anthropology professor was just here." This was stated as though my presence was quite unusual. Kevin went on to say, "Yeah, I invited her." That would have been an interesting conversation to witness. At that point in time, I had a hard time going anywhere and not bumping into a former student.

Kevin went on to complete his Exploration Project on suspension arts. His presentations were excellent, and the master of ceremonies came to class with Kevin on the day of his in-class presentation and open house and assisted Kevin with his presentations, explaining the logistics of suspension performance and his many roles. Despite Kevin's apprehensions, he had a completely captive audience during both presentations. Students were perhaps more interested in Kevin's work than any other project presented that day. It was excellent.

Ramirez said: "[y]ou can neither 'read' yourself nor 'think' yourself into competence on issues of diversity; when it comes to diversity, self-invention requires a willingness to 'experience.'"[22] Indeed, I had experienced diversity. I had come into solidarity with Kevin, and I learned a lot about myself and the culture of suspension arts. I taught at the community college from the fall of 2006 to the spring of 2011.

Prior to this teaching experience, I knew very little about community colleges and their students. Most of what I did know was inaccurate. My father attended a community college when I was very young, and that was the only frame of reference I had up until the time I began teaching. Teaching at the community college was intensely rewarding. I met and worked with a very wide variety of students. And since then, I have been in a continuous process of building solidarity with students.

## REFLECTIONS ON AN AGED VIGNETTE

Experiences like the one above concretized for me an interconnected career pathway and research agenda. While working as an adjunct instructor at the community college, I was also pursuing a doctoral degree. Upon completing that degree, and for the past 10-plus years, I have been working as a professor at a four-year institution preparing students to become leaders within higher education. I routinely interact with graduate students at the master's and doctoral level.

While only a handful of these students have a keen interest in the community college space, I frame understanding this sector of higher education as critical for all. I teach all the community college-related courses at my current home institution and make significant use of stories as course content and pedagogy.[23] Teaching at the community college instilled in me a passion for the students and faculty at these institutions—it served as the impetus for my doctoral dissertation, wherein I sought to understand how community college students construct their educational lives, as well as my past, current, and future research.

The above vignette provides a look into my recollection of a singular event I experienced as a community college faculty member. Elements of my pedagogy, commitment to students, willingness to learn and experience, identities, and personhood come through here, or at least that is the intent and hope. Solidarity with students is important to me as an undergirding element of a pedagogy I view as relational, feminist, critical, and liberatory.[24]

Understanding students—something I consistently aspire toward, both then and now—can mean unlearning, suspending and critiquing beliefs, and experiencing discomfort, anxiety, and fear. By showing up for Kevin and navigating a space comfortable to him but not me, at least at the beginning, we engaged in a de facto bidirectional socialization process.[25] He learned from me, and I learned from him. We impressed upon each other as well as the microculture of our classroom space that semester.

As how many students may feel, the community college classroom space may not have been the most comfortable environment for Kevin. When I started teaching at the community college, I became quickly and keenly aware that many students were not quick to trust me or my intentions, the result of years experiencing educational spaces as punitive, hurtful, and generally negative. And at the same time, that bar scene was not a familiar or comfortable space to me.

Those impressions, feelings, and comfort levels changed for both of us, and solidarity grew up around us. Kevin certainly learned more from that solidarity than from being questioned by another instructor who conflated engaging in suspension arts and psychological problems, which was wholly invalidating.

While this vignette and this reflection may not have immediately apparent connections to the topic at hand, writing myself into this book will help readers understand my positionality; who I am as a teacher and person is inextricably connected to who I am as a researcher. Knowing me will help readers understand my sense-making process, which has led to the development of this work. This premise (knowing me is understanding my sense-making) and these connections (pedagogy is related to inquiry) will become more and more apparent throughout the book.

## WHO I AM AND WHO I AM NOT

In terms of my identities, I identify as a white, queer, middle-aged, cisgender (though I am sometimes read as androgenous) woman. Having shared racial and gender identities with most participants in this study certainly affected the data and my interpretation of it, though the nature of those effects was difficult to discern at points. More on this is forthcoming. As I have worked on this project, onlookers have made sundry assumptions about me as a researcher interested in understanding how community college faculty make sense of their students' mental health.

It must be noted that I am not a psychologist, counselor, or mental health professional of any kind. I have not been trained in nor have I had any formal training related to mental health. Yet, I know community college faculty, and I know community college students. This book is not about diagnosing mental illness; it is not about treating mental illness. It is about knowing faculty and students. My knowing comes from experience, previous inquiries, interfacing with the relevant literature, and engaging with community college faculty as part of carrying out the study upon which this book is based.

That I do not have a background in psychology, counseling, or mental health does not preclude me from writing about it. Most of the faculty I interviewed for this study had no formal experience or background with mental health, yet we were able to speak about it candidly, fluidly, and competently within the context of their experiences with students. Again, this text is not about diagnosing or treating mental illness. This is a book about community college faculty and students and has a specific focus on students' mental health.

## ORGANIZATION OF THE BOOK

This chapter is followed by four sections, housing ten chapters (11 total chapters). Appendices are included, which highlight the study's conceptual framework wherein I outline elements of the epistemology, methodology, methods, and data analysis.

The first section, entitled *The Background*, houses two chapters. The first chapter in this section, *Community College Faculty and their Students*, is framed as one part commentary and one part literature review to acquaint readers with community college faculty and their students. While largely attending to the extant literature, I also infuse this and some subsequent chapters with my personal experiences as a community college faculty member—as well as the research I have done with these educators.

The second chapter within this section, *Research on Community College Student Mental Health*, provides readers with a comprehensive account of what is already known about community college student mental health. I frame 2015 as a key momentum point and lay out the events that spurred an increased interest in this topic. While the body of literature in this area remains underdeveloped and is still growing, the information shared within this chapter gives a solid foundation for the remainder of the book.

The second section of the book, *The Faculty*, contains two chapters. During the interviews, I spent a lot of time talking with the participants about their faculty lives. I introduce the study's participants in the first of these chapters, *Career Pathways, Dispositions, and Pedagogies* by discussing their career pathways, professional dispositions, and pedagogical approaches. Faculty said much about their students' assets and challenges regarding college-going. Resiliency and poverty will be a major focus of the second of these chapters, *Students' Assets and Obstacles*, as these were framed as students' biggest asset and biggest obstacle.

The third section of the book, *The Discussions*, contains four chapters and is focused on the thematic strands of the interviews I conducted. The first chapter in this section is entitled *Doing Emotional Labor*. Faculty involved in this study engaged in significant emotional labor as a normative underpinning of their work as pedagogues. Within this chapter, I overlay evidence of this with a gender-centered lens. Nearly all participants engaged in what I viewed as a care-centered, affect-conscious, and feminist approach to teaching. Furthermore, all but three participants identified as women. That only three man-identifying persons volunteered for the study is of considerable note.

Within the second chapter of this section, *Rejecting the Monolith*, I challenge the notion that all community college students navigating through a mental health issue are the same. Faculty expressed a rich and nuanced view of their students as it relates to mental health. Here I present a perceptual typology of students co-built within and from my conversations with faculty. This typology is framed as a useful mental model, which discourages thinking about students in a monolithic fashion.

*Navigating Institutional Structures and Systems* is the title of the third chapter in this section. Faculty discussed frustrations in navigating institutional structures and systems related to supporting students with mental health concerns. The lack of feedback provided after referring students to the institution's behavioral intervention team was highlighted as a particular challenge. There were also concerns about the potential for college personnel to equate a student mental health concern with trouble or emergency.

The final chapter within this section is titled, *Making It Work*. Faculty explained a broad palette of ways they supported students with mental health concerns. These conversations included more than just strategies. We discussed ways of seeing students, ways of approaching the classroom space, and ways of being present for and in the presence of students.

The fourth and final section of the book, *The Future*, contains two chapters. Within the first chapter, *What Can We Do Now?*, I outline what can be done now as it relates to the insights gleaned from these faculty and the literature, while also taking into account the current and future shape of the contexts within which this issue exists. By taking into account the first nine chapters of the book, I provide practical ways community colleges can start the process of better serving students who are managing or trying to manage a mental health issue—diagnosed or not.

Rather than take a one size fits all approach, I attend to the nuance of each institution that must be considered. While the findings of this study were never meant to be broadly generalized, they do provide many points of consideration for all community colleges. The final chapter of the book is called, *How Might the Future Look?,* and in keeping with the focus of the Futures Series on Community Colleges, the series of which this book is a part, here I consider the possible futures that community colleges could choose to pursue to successfully support students in light of the mental health concerns they may be facing.

Mental health is and will continue to be a concern on community college campuses for the foreseeable future. If student support and success are embedded into any given community college's values or mission statement, this issue must be acknowledged, assessed, addressed, and redressed. Without being prescriptive, I lay out ideas about what this might look like.

## SUMMARY

Within this introductory chapter, I provided readers with an overview of the issue this book addresses. In short, community college student mental health is a major concern among community college leaders, as it affects students' educational lives. Poor mental health can have negative effects on myriad student success measures such as grades, GPA, persistence, and completion. Community college students have more instances of and more severe mental health issues than their four-year institution counterparts and have less access to resources and support.

I also shared an overview of the study that inspired and generated much fodder for this text. In doing so, my positionality as a researcher, writer, pedagogue, interpreter, knower, and knowledge creator is provided. This allows readers to better understand the perspective from which this work was conceived of, built, and put forward. My background as a deep insider is explained.

To close the chapter, I gave an overview of what is to follow within the book. The total text contains eleven chapters, this one included. What follows includes four sections that house 10 chapters. This book was written from a place of deep respect for community college faculty and students. I consistently marvel at the skillful teaching and deep learning that happens within our nation's community colleges day in and day out. My hope is that this book provides readers with an understanding of the extant research, the study I conducted, and what steps can be taken to address and begin to redress this profound issue and stark reality.

## NOTES

1. Brenda G. Kucirka, "Navigating the Faculty-Student Relationship: Interacting with Nursing Students with Mental Health Issues," *Journal of the American Psychiatric Nurses Association* 23, no. 6 (November/December 2017): 393–403, https://doi.org/10.1177/1078390317705451.

2. See Amanda O. Latz, "Flow in the Community College Classroom?: An Autoethnographic Exploration," *International Journal for the Scholarship of Teaching and Learning* 6, no. 2 (2012): 1–13, http://digitalcommons.georgiasouthern.edu/ij-sotl/vol6/iss2/15/.

3. Regina Deil-Amen, "Socio-Academic Integrative Moments: Rethinking Academic and Social Integration among Two-Year College Students in Career-Related Programs," *The Journal of Higher Education* 82 no. 1 (2011): 54–91, https://doi.org/10.1080/00221546.2011.11779085; Amanda O. Latz, "Understanding Community College Student Persistence through Photovoice: An Emergent Model," *Journal of College Student Retention: Research, Theory & Practice* 16, no. 4 (February 2015): 487–509. https://doi.org/10.2190/CS.16.4.b.

4. Vincent Tinto, *Leaving College: Rethinking the Causes and Cures of Student Attrition*, 2nd ed. (Chicago: University of Chicago Press, 1993).

5. Laura I. Rendón, "Validating Culturally Diverse Students: Toward a New Model of Learning and Student Development," *Innovative Higher Education* 19 (September 1994): 33–51, https://doi.org/10.1007/BF01191156.

6. Deil-Amen, "Socio-Academic Integrative Moments."

7. Lauren Schudde, "Short- and Long-term Impacts of Engagement Experiences with Faculty and Peers at Community Colleges," *Review of Higher Education* 42 (Winter 2019): 385–426, https://doi.org/10.1353/rhe.2019.0001.

8. Jennifer M. Cadigan, Jennifer C. Duckworth, and Christine M. Lee, "Physical and Mental Health Issues Facing Community College Students," *Journal of American College Health* 70, no. 3 (2020): 891–897, http://doi.org/10.1080/07448481.2020.1776716; Thomas N. Hollins, "Student Life and Student Engagement Programs and Services in the Community College," in *Handbook for Student Affairs in Community Colleges*, eds. Ashley Tull, Linda Kuk, and Paulette Dalpes (Sterling, VA: Stylus, 2015), 218–38.

9. Daniel Eisenberg et al., *Too Distressed to Learn? Mental Health among Community College Students* (Washington, DC: ACCT), https://www.acct.org/product/too-distressed-learn-mental-health-among-community-college-students-2016; Sarah Ketchen Lipson et al., "Mental Health Conditions Among Community College Students: A National Study of Prevalence and Use of Treatment Services," *Psychiatric Services* 72, no. 10 (October 2021): 1126–1133, https://doi.org/10.1176/appi.ps.202000437

10. Daniel Seth Katz and Karen Davison, "Community College Student Mental Health: A Comparative Analysis," *Community College Review* 42, no. 4 (October 2014): 307–26, https://doi.org/10.1177/0091552114535466.

11. Alan M. Schwitzer and Brian Van Brunt, "Student Mental Health Issues on Today's Campuses," in *Today's College Students: A Reader*, eds. Pietro A. Sasso and Joseph. L. DeVitis (New York: Peter Lang, 2015): 331–45.

12. Schwitzer and Van Brunt, "Student Mental Health."

13. Schwitzer and Van Brunt, "Student Mental Health," 341.

14. Paula E. McBride, "Addressing the Lack of Mental Health Services for At-Risk Students at a Two-Year Community College: A Contemporary Review," *Community College Journal of Research and Practice* 43, no. 2 (2019), 147 (my italics), https://doi.org/10.1080/10668926.2017.1409670.

15. Katharine J. Herbert, Amy Baize-Ward, and Amanda O. Latz, "Transformative Pedagogy with Innovative Methodology: Using Photovoice to Understand Community College Student Needs," *Community College Journal of Research and Practice* 42, no. 7–8, 536–549, https://doi.org/10.1080/10668926.2018.1431572.

16. Schudde, "Short- and Long-Term Impacts."

17. Alan M. Schwitzer and John A. Vaughn, "Mental Health, Well-Being, and Learning: Supporting Our Students in Times of Need," *About Campus* 22, no. 20 (May/June 2017), 4–11. https://doi.org/10.1002/abc.21287.

18. Herbert, Baize-Ward, and Latz, "Transformative Pedagogy."

19. Virginia Braun and Victoria Clarke, *Thematic Analysis: A Practical Guide* (Thousand Oaks, CA: Sage, 2022).

20. Yvonne S. Lincoln and Egon G. Guba, *Naturalistic Inquiry* (Newbury Park, CA: Sage, 1985).

21. Mihaly Csikszentmihalyi, *Flow: The Psychology of Optimal Experience* (New York: HarperCollins, 1990).

22. Blandina Cardenas Ramirez, "Creating a New Kind of Leadership for Campus Diversity," in *Organization and Governance in Higher Education*, 5th ed., ed. M. Christopher Brown (Boston, MA: Pearson, 2000): 406–414.

23. See Amanda O. Latz and Keri L. Rodgers, "Photovoice and Visual Life Writing: Infusing Participant Research into Graduate Pedagogy," in *Engaging Images: Utilizing Visuals to Understand and Promote Student Development Research, Pedagogy, and Practice*, eds. Bridget Turner Kelly and Carrie A. Kortegast (Sterling, VA: Stylus, 2018): 91–104.

24. bell hooks, *Teaching to Transgress: Education as the Practice of Freedom* (New York: Routledge, 1994); Amanda O. Latz, "Flow in the Community College Classroom?: An Autoethnographic Exploration," *International Journal for the Scholarship of Teaching and Learning* 6, no. 2 (2012): 1–13, http://digitalcommons.georgiasouthern.edu/ij-sotl/vol6/iss2/15/.

25. Robert A. Rhoads and James R. Valadez, *Democracy, Multiculturalism, and the Community College: A Critical Perspective* (New York: Garland, 1996).

# PART I

# The Background

Before diving into the details of the study upon which this book is based, background information on community college faculty, community college students, and community college student mental health is provided. This background information clarifies the context within which the study was conducted and summarizes what is known about the topic based on the scholarly literature and other sources.

Community college faculty can play a major role in the educational lives of their students, and many do. The work context, demography, preparation and professional development, work conditions, employment status, and experiences and impact of this unique faculty group are highlighted within chapter 2. This chapter is also threaded through with information on community college students and the community college sector in general.

Chapter 3 is focused community college student mental health research. Prior to 2015, there was almost no literature on this topic. But in 2015, largely in response to the mass shooting that took place at Umpqua Community College, this literature body began to grow. While it is inaccurate and irresponsible to conflate mental health issues and violence, this event gained national attention and placed community college student mental health in the spotlight. And while what is known still lacks in comparison to the four-year sector, a lot of good work has been done during the interceding years. It is laid out in detail within chapter 3.

# Chapter 2

# Community College Faculty and their Students

"I like, really, just getting to interact with our students."

–Tess

"There's this amazing panorama of society [within the student body]."

–Carolyn

Community college faculty are at the core of carrying out the institution's academic mission. These individuals play a significant role in a student's experience at the college and have the potential to change students' lives. Many community college faculty know community college students very well; interviews conducted as part of this book project suggest some community college faculty are *students* of their students. This is a good thing, as "[f]aculty knowledge of student populations can improve instruction."[1]

Knowing students can give way to insights about how to teach, how to create an environment conducive to learning, and how to build relationships inside the learning space. Because much of the content of this text is derived from interviews with community college faculty, it is important to provide an overview of this faculty cadre. This chapter will be partitioned into the following sections: work context; demography; preparation and professional development; work conditions; employment status, impact on students; and community college faculty and student mental health.

## WORK CONTEXT

Whereas the blueprints for the first higher education institutions in the United States came from England and Germany, the community college concept is unique to the United States. Like most inventions, the community college was created for and has been continuously charged with solving problems. Most recently, this means preparing individuals for an increasingly complex workplace—requiring critical thinking, problem-solving skills, and the ability to work collaboratively.

At the start of the twentieth century, the nature of work in the United States was in a change process—moving farther away from an agrarian economy and more toward an industrialized one. Work required more education, and more people were entering work. Therefore, more people required some level of postsecondary education. Indeed, the community college context has changed considerably since its inception in 1901 with the creation of Joliet Junior College.

These institutions were born from the secondary sector. They were originally meant to alleviate some of the burdens of extant four-year institutions by focusing on the first two years of college, leaving the four-year institutions to pour their efforts into the upper division. However, the four-year sector never let go of the first two years.

Faculty work at the community college was centered on teaching, not the production of research or the pursuit of external funding to support research endeavors. The fingerprints of the colleges' inception remain today. For example, some community colleges are partially funded through local taxes, service districts are often clearly delineated with geo-political demarcations, and faculty are still largely focused on teaching while not being expected to carry out research.

The Truman Commission Report, published in 1947, provided an expanded and more inclusive vision for higher education, in which education and democracy are seen as intertwined. The important role of the community college within the United States was concretized through this document, which articulated the sector as an "agent for change, liberation, and hope in communities across the nation."[2]

On the heels of the report, the community college landscape in the United States exploded in the 1960s and 1970s to account for the Baby Boomer generation post-World War II and the ongoing expansion of the industrialization of work and the rise of the global marketplace. During this period, the organization and oversight of community colleges began to resemble what it looks like today. State-level coordination of the states' higher education offerings began to take shape.

For example, the California Master Plan outlined the state's three-tiered system, which included California Community Colleges, The California State University, and The University of California. This plan brought the state's postsecondary education efforts into a unified whole with a common set of policies, language, and traversal mechanism for students.

This period also marked significant progress for civil rights activists within the country, making higher education more accessible for persons from low-income backgrounds, women, and Black, Indigenous, Hispanic/Latinx/a/o, Asian, and other persons with marginalized racial/ethnic identities (these are not exclusive categories). Many community colleges that exist today were born of this growth period.

According to the American Association of Community Colleges,[3] there are presently 1,043 community colleges throughout the United States; this includes 936 public, 35 tribal, and 72 independent colleges. In the fall of 2020, these institutions enrolled (headcount) a total of 10.3 million students, with 6.2 million in the credit-earning curriculum and 4.1 million in the non-credit space. This number of students equates to 39 percent of all undergraduate students in the United States.

Some of the largest community colleges enroll well over 40,000 students at any given time. Examples include Houston Community College, Northern Virginia Community College, and Miami Dade College. On the other hand, some enroll fewer than 100, such as Keweenaw Bay Ojibwa Community College in Michigan and Deep Springs College in Nevada. Approximately 28 percent of community colleges offer on-campus student housing, often a feature of rural institutions and those with significant student-athlete and international student populations. The average enrollment at associate degree–granting institutions is roughly 6,300 students.[4]

Community colleges play a significant role in the overall higher education landscape within the United States. Of note, among those bachelor's degree holders who graduated between 2008 and 2017, over half (52%) earned at least some credit from a community college. This is a slight increase in comparison to previous years. And one-fourth of those who earned a bachelor's degree also earned an associate's degree along the way.[5]

Community colleges are often known for their access imperative. They are much more affordable than four-year institutions, at just over one-third of the cost. During 2021–2022, the average annual tuition and fees for a community college was $3,800, whereas it was $10,740 at public four-year institutions.[6]

Nearly any person within the United States can access the community college for a wide range of resources, which may include daycare and summer programming for children; dual or concurrent enrollment or credit programs for middle and high school students; associate's degrees that lead to transfer to four-year institutions; (applied) bachelor's degrees (in some but not all states; typically limited in scope and focused on high demand subject areas); applied associate's degrees that lead directly to work but also leave the door to transfer open; subassociate's credentials that can lead to work or be stacked into a degree; noncredit learning opportunities and credentials; a few summer courses to augment the curriculum at a four-year institution; English language learning; GED preparation; workout and recreation facilities; and lifelong learning courses such as watercolor painting, produce canning, or tax preparation. Both a strength and a weakness of community colleges, they are known for their multiple missions and their attempt to be all things for all people.[7]

In line with their access mission, admissions criteria at community colleges are typically minimal, and help is available to prospective students during the admissions process. Most students who apply are admitted to the institution; however, admittance to the institution does not equate to admission to all academic programs.

Some academic programs are highly selective and low in numbers. Nursing, sonography, and dental hygiene are some examples. If an admitted student does not have evidence of past academic achievement or ability (i.e., high school transcript, standardized test scores), many institutions will require students to take placement tests in the areas of reading, writing, and math to determine at what level that student should begin coursework. This practice is typically relegated to the credit-bearing course space. Sometimes, that means a student will be placed into developmental courses, which will not count toward their eventual credential.

Therefore, while the community college is considered open access, that access is only applied to the front door. Access narrows once inside. This means community college faculty are encountering and working with a very wide variety of students. For each faculty member, the width of the spectrum of students they teach depends on where they are situated within the college. Those who teach courses without any prerequisites may see a very broad array of students, while those teaching selective programs within the allied health areas, for example, will see a narrow slice of that group.

As noted earlier, the comprehensive community college is known for its multiple missions, which include transfer education; career, technical, and workforce education; developmental education; and community education. These are not discrete categories, however. Students enrolled in developmental education courses may concurrently take courses that are part of the transfer curriculum, and students engaged in community education may also be part of a workforce development initiative.

The faculty work context within each of these components of a comprehensive community college mission is very different. For example, a full-time culinary arts faculty member may spend three days of the week teaching groups of students within a kitchen laboratory for hours at a time.

To contrast, a part-time faculty member who teaches one section of a developmental math course online may never step foot on campus and interact with students only through the institution's learning management system (LMS), email, and video conferencing platform. In another example, a local watercolor artist may be asked to teach a series of art classes at the college during the summer, such as *Wine and Watercolor*, and be paid a modest stipend for each class. Again, the work context for each of these instructors is very different, and those differences are often mediated by which part(s) of the mission their teaching work is meant to fulfill.

Most of the community college faculty I have come to know over the years share a common characteristic: they love teaching and are excellent teachers. When you routinely work alongside students with markedly different backgrounds, a wide variety of identities, and varying levels of academic ability, you must be creative to be successful. In some ways, teaching within the community college can feel like teaching in a one-room schoolhouse— you must continuously adapt and adjust so all students can learn and make gains in their burgeoning understandings of course concepts, critical thinking abilities, and skills acquisition. With the recent explosion of dual enrollment, concurrent enrollment, and dual credit options for secondary students, age ranges in any given community college classroom could conceivably range from as young as 11 (grade six) to 80 years old or older.

Imagine teaching a class that includes an early teenager who is still uncertain about their intended career path and a person in their 70s who recently retired. This is quite a unique challenge. As noted by Gail Mellow and Cynthia Heelan, "[t]he greatest challenge for community colleges is embracing and supporting the most diverse classroom of students ever to sit side by side in American higher education."[8] Community college faculty are at the center of this challenge.

Community college students are characterized by their diversity and significant numbers.[9] Again, there are over 10 million community college students in the United States—6.2 million are credit seeking, and 4.1 million are pursuing educational opportunities within the noncredit sphere.[10]

Of those seeking college credit, only 35 percent are enrolled full-time and 60 percent are women. Forty-four percent are white, 27 percent are Hispanic, 12 percent are Black, 7 percent are Asian or Pacific Islander, 1 percent are Native American, 4 percent are two or more races, 4 percent identified as other or unknown, and 1 percent are nonresident aliens.[11] Community colleges serve the majority of Native American and Hispanic college students. The average age is 27, while the median age is 23.[12]

The diversity of individuals who access this sector of higher education is significant and unparalleled. Many are parenting, and 15 percent are single parents. Some are engaging in elder care. Nearly one-third are first-generation college students. Eight percent are non-US citizens, and 4 percent are veterans. Eight percent of community college students have a bachelor's degree, and 20 percent have a disability. Community college students often juggle many roles in addition to being students. For example, 62 percent of full-time students and 72 percent of part-time students are working in addition to taking college courses.[13]

Many community college students are living in poverty. In the past few years, scholars have focused on unmet basic needs among community college students.[14] The data are striking.

Basic needs insecurity includes food and housing insecurity as well as a lack of access to mental health support. As many as 61 percent of community college students may be experiencing basic needs insecurity.[15] Furthermore, those students with basic needs insecurity are more likely to have mental health issues than their resource-secure peers.[16] The COVID-19 global pandemic exacerbated this issue.

## FACULTY DEMOGRAPHY

In 2020, approximately 281,030 faculty were employed by two-year degree-granting institutions of higher education in the United States.[17] Locating accurate national data on the demography of community college faculty is difficult. It is also unwieldy because of the significant proportion of part-time faculty, a necessarily transitory group from one term to the next. In terms of gender and race, though, community college faculty are mostly women and overwhelmingly white.[18]

Approximately 70 percent of faculty at community colleges are employed part-time.[19] Because part-time (also known as adjunct or contingent) faculty are typically employed through short-term or semester-based contracts, their numbers are constantly in flux. Their proportionality to full-time faculty, however, will likely remain steady or increase over time as colleges continue to enact cost-saving strategies amid enrollment fluctuations and an unsteady public funding landscape, especially in light of the pandemic.[20]

## PREPARATION AND PROFESSIONAL DEVELOPMENT

Most community college faculty hold a master's degree. Some hold credentials appropriate for their subject area and similar to a master's degree. Like the four-year sector, faculty credentials are important, especially in terms of accreditation. Faculty are expected to be subject matter experts. Unlike the secondary sector, however, community college faculty are not required to hold any sort of credentials or licensing related to teaching. And some may enter their teaching positions not knowing anything about the community college environment.

Because graduate education often occurs within research universities, faculty socialization within graduate school does not prepare individuals to work within a diverse variety of postsecondary institutions such as the community college.[21] In fact, some may harbor negative attitudes about the community college after being socialized within a graduate program on the campus of a four-year institution.

Because of these factors—and because ongoing professional learning is necessary regardless of position or place of work—most community college faculty are encouraged and sometimes required or incentivized to engage in professional development throughout their careers. Professional development for community college faculty occurs on many levels and on many topics. It can be long- or short-term.

Faculty may engage in professional development on their own (individual), through the offerings of their institution (institutional), or through four-year institutions or external professional organizations (organizational). Individual-level professional development may include reading; testing out new teaching strategies, activities, or assessments; enrolling in a massive, open, online course (MOOC); listening to podcasts; watching videos and documentaries; seeking certifications (e.g., Mental Health First Aid); and engaging on professional learning platforms such as Udemy and LinkedIn Learning.

Institutional-level professional development may include on-campus workshops, campus-sponsored book clubs, in-service learning days, grow-your-own leadership programs, and online faculty learning communities. Organizational-level professional development may include leadership workshops, annual conferences, and webinars. Many community college faculty also pursue doctoral education in their subject area or in the discipline of community college leadership.

## WORK CONDITIONS

Teaching within the community college is quite different from teaching within a four-year institution. Full-time faculty teach four or five classes in any given term, typically carrying a higher course load than faculty at four-year institutions. Because of the nature of the curricula, these faculty are usually teaching developmental-, 100-, and/or 200-level courses. Courses generally consist of traditional lectures, laboratories, and/or supervision of field or clinical experiences. Courses are offered in a face-to-face, online, and/or blended format. The COVID-19 pandemic also ushered in the Hyflex classroom, where some students may be in person while others attend virtually while still others may watch the recorded session later.[22]

Class sizes at community colleges tend to be smaller than at four-year institutions. While lecture halls filled with hundreds of students are commonplace at many universities across the country, it is quite rare to see a class larger than 30 or 40 students at a community college. Depending on the college and work expectations, full-time faculty at community colleges may also engage in activities such as advising students, sitting on various committees, scheduling courses, revising curricula, serving as a faculty advisor for a student group, recruiting and orienting part-time faculty, and participating in accreditation activities, which may include program review, assessment of student learning outcomes, and report writing.

Community college faculty are not usually incentivized to conduct and publish research in the same way faculty at four-year institutions often are. Teaching is paramount at the community college. This does not, however, preclude community college faculty from being scholars. Some are quite active within the research communities connected with their field, and some even seek external funding for research projects.

It is also important to note that teaching can be a scholarly pursuit. There is an entire field termed the Scholarship of Teaching and Learning (SoTL), wherein the classroom, broadly defined, is seen as a site of inquiry. Many community college faculty engage in dedicated pedagogical development and improvement by systematically interrogating their own teaching practice. This is evident within scholarly outlets such as the journal *Teaching English in the Two-Year College*, published by the National Council of Teachers of English.

Related to the general lack of incentivization of research within the community college sphere is the community college context itself. Faculty at four-year institutions often have scaffolding in place for their work, such as teaching assistants (upper-level students working with lower-level students), graduate programs that can support graduate assistantships, laboratory spaces, psychology undergraduates eager (or required) to participate in studies, and entire offices dedicated to helping secure external funding for research projects. This kind of scaffolding does not exist within the community college space—at least not to the same degree.

Community colleges do not typically have upper-level students, graduate programs, graduate assistantships, laboratory spaces conducive to research, large psychology departments, or extensive support for securing research funding. Moreover, many community college faculty are trained at the master's level—or an equivalent credential dependent on their field. Without a doctoral degree, which in many cases is designed to train independent researchers, those faculty who are master's-trained may not have the skills or desire necessary to maintain an active research agenda and record of scholarly output.

This is a changing and ever-evolving landscape, however. Community colleges were born from secondary schools, which is from where the teaching focus derives. Yet, as community colleges' missions shift and boundaries are spanned, so does faculty work. For example, the community college baccalaureate is a force driving different kinds of faculty work, some in the direction of research activity. In addition, Montgomery College's Germantown Campus in Maryland boasts an on-campus hospital. Having a hospital on campus offers a wellspring of innovative teaching and clinical education opportunities—as well as research activity and grant-seeking efforts.

Most community college faculty are satisfied with their jobs. There are certainly challenging aspects of the work, however. It can be difficult for newer faculty to adjust to the varying levels of their students' academic experiences and preparedness. It can be startling, for example, to realize that one or more students in your class may be functionally illiterate.

In addition, most community college students are part-time.[23] Many hold and manage an entire set of disparate roles, each with high stakes obligations. Newer faculty may be surprised with how students' employment, childcare needs, and unreliable transportation can lead to frequent absences, incomplete work, and even attrition. While some community colleges do offer honors programs and classes, developmental education is more commonplace. Developmental courses, which are typically offered in the areas of reading, writing, and math, are not typically the most desirable courses to teach.

Furthermore, sometimes social class differences between faculty and students serve as a foundation for miscommunication at a fundamental level. Full-time community college faculty, who are typically highly educated and firmly middle class, may struggle to fully understand the lived experiences of many of their students who are living in poverty.[24] Despite this, there are plentiful opportunities at the community college level to make a significant difference in students' lives.

Many faculty love having the opportunity to work with an extremely diverse student body—while it may be challenging, it can also be immensely rewarding. There are opportunities to literally change students' lives on a regular basis. Faculty also often recognize and praise students' resiliency. Many students arrive to classroom spaces having defied multiple odds stacked against them such as negative secondary education experiences, addiction, abuse, and various forms of marginalization and oppression. That they have even stepped foot on campus, or logged into the institution's learning management system, is often a triumph in and of itself.

Affordances and conditions surrounding employment as a full-time faculty member at the community college level vary significantly across both states and institutions. Because each state's community college landscape, including history, mission, governance, funding, and accountability, varies significantly,[25] so do the work conditions for faculty. Tenure does exist within the community college sector, but to a lesser extent than at four-year institutions. Additionally, unions and collective bargaining are variably available and/or legal depending on contexts. Opportunities to participate in shared governance also vary significantly.

## PART-TIME FACULTY

It is critical to highlight that a significant majority of community college faculty are part-time. These adjunct, or contingent, faculty members are vast in number, and community colleges simply could not function without them. That said, this faculty group is too often overlooked, underappreciated, and insufficiently paid.

For example, in the fall of 2020, the adjusted nine-month salary for full-time instructional staff at community colleges was $67,313.[26] To contrast, the majority of adjunct faculty across all institution types make $3500 or less per class.[27] Teaching 10 community college classes as an adjunct at $3500 per class would earn $35,000. And this stipend would typically come without health insurance, retirement benefits, or job security. Yet some adjunct faculty have full-time employment elsewhere.

When considering adjunct faculty, it is important to actively reject monolithic thinking about this key group. Simply put, not all adjunct faculty are the same. Judith Gappa and David Leslie built a helpful typology of part-time faculty members.[28] First, *aspiring academics* are part-time faculty whose career goal is to secure full-time employment as a faculty member. These faculty members are often teaching multiple courses at multiple institutions while concurrently pursuing doctoral degrees and/or actively applying for full-time positions. This part-time faculty group is often highlighted when concerns around low-wages, short-term contracts, abysmal job prospects, lack of representation in shared governance, and limited access to benefits of any kind are raised.

Next are *career enders*. These part-time faculty members are on the opposite end of the career lifecycle; they are working less while maintaining some involvement in the working world. These are individuals who, for example, may be moving away from full-time teaching or a full-time career in a specific field (e.g., accounting, nursing). Career enders teach because they want to give back, enjoy the classroom, or are filling a distinct need any given community college may have.

The third type are *specialists* or *professionals*. These faculty members have niche expertise in a particular area that positions them as aptly qualified to teach certain subjects. An example may be the head brew master at a local brewery teaching a course in fermentation science. These faculty usually have a full-time job in their field and teach part-time because they enjoy teaching and interacting with students.

The last type are *freelancers*. These faculty members make a living by putting together multiple part-time employment opportunities and often work based on short-term contracts going from project to project. An example is a freelance writer who regularly contributes to several outlets while also advancing book-length projects. Someone in a position like this one may teach a course in creative writing or developmental English.

While not part of this original typology, which was created in 1993, but relevant today is the *exclusively online* adjunct faculty member who may be teaching at multiple institutions all across the country (or world) in an online format. These online adjuncts may be place-bound for various reasons and/or particularly skilled in online pedagogies.

## FACULTY IMPACT ON STUDENTS

Generally, student interaction with community college faculty has positive outcomes for students. The results of Lundberg's study suggested faculty-student interaction inside and outside the classroom is beneficial for community college students.[29] Frequent interaction with faculty predicted gains in general education, intellectual skills, science and technology, personal development, and career preparation. Therefore, "[c]ommunity colleges must continue to identify ways to foster and reward faculty interaction with students."[30]

More recent research corroborated these findings. Lauren Schudde found that "academic engagement with [community college] faculty outside of class offers positive returns for both short- and long-term college outcomes."[31] Academic interactions between community college students and faculty are especially important considering "community college students are indeed less likely to engage with members of the campus community outside of the classroom than their four-year counterparts."[32] Because most community colleges are commuter institutions, this makes sense. Intentional efforts to encourage more student-faculty interactions will only benefit student success.

Upon disaggregating student course withdrawal data, leaders at Odessa College realized these rates varied based on instructors even when accounting for other potential mediating factors.[33] The follow-up question was: Why? Leaders at this institution sought to answer this key question.

After carrying out classroom observations and faculty interviews, it was determined that faculty interactions with students, or positive *faculty-student relationships*, made all the difference. Key factors related to course persistence were leveraged into a program meant to build faculty-student relationships: learning students' names in week one, being current on student course progress and intervening when needed, meeting and sharing feedback with students routinely, and having strong course structure while allowing for some flexibility.[3434]

## COMMUNITY COLLEGE FACULTY AND STUDENT MENTAL HEALTH

Given their impact on students, faculty may be playing an increasingly key part in student mental health because of the pandemic. In fact, a recent report from Sarah Ketchen Lipson, Amber Talaski, and Nina Cesare was premised on this idea.[35]

Key findings of their study included that 87 percent of faculty believe student mental health worsened during the COVID-19 pandemic, and 80 percent of faculty have had outreach conversations with students about mental health. Half of faculty reported having a good idea of when a student is in emotional or mental distress, and 73 percent of faculty want more professional development on student mental health. The majority (61%) of faculty thought training on student mental health should be mandatory. And, finally, 21 percent of faculty believe supporting students with mental health issues has taken a toll on their own mental health.

While there is some literature regarding the perceptions and experiences faculty have of and with students with mental health issues, most of this research is set within the four-year sector. Yet much of that literature is relevant and transferrable to the community college sector—with some caveats. Because this book is shaped by interviews with community college faculty about the mental health of their students, what is known based on the four-year sector is included here and segmented into four subsections: faculty awareness and perceptions of student mental health, comfortability and confidence, influencing factors, and recommendations.

## Faculty Awareness and Perceptions of Student Mental Health

In 2001, Kelsey Backels and Inese Wheeler stated "[f]aculty perceptions of the effect of mental health issues on academic functioning have not been studied."[36] That has since changed to some degree. Most faculty members in Backel and Wheeler's study viewed mental health issues as influencing students' academic performance.[37]

The only problem not seen as affecting academic performance by a majority of faculty in Backel and Wheeler's study were gay, lesbian, or bisexuality concerns.[38] It should be noted that this study was conducted over two decades ago, and much has changed since that time (e.g., passing of the Marriage Equality Act). However, most respondents would extend flexibility for the following problems: death of a parent, family problem, learning disability, rape or sexual assault, depression, and suicidal ideation.

Another study on this topic, conducted by Marion Becker and colleagues in 2002, included both faculty members and students at the University of South Florida.[39] Two-thirds of faculty (65%) viewed themselves as able to discuss their concerns about students exhibiting mental health concerns, while only 40 percent of students viewed themselves able to do so.

Most faculty (68%) in Becker et al.'s study were very familiar with available mental health services, though students were not.[40] Notably, 73 percent of students reported being very *unfamiliar* with university resources. Faculty who reported being very familiar with resources were more likely to refer students to those resources. In addition, half of the faculty reported not feeling comfortable working with a student with mental illness; 10 percent reported they would feel very uncomfortable.

## Comfortability and Confidence

While many community college faculty may know how to help students managing mental health concerns, they may not be comfortable or confident in doing so. K. L. Margrove et al. found that 62.6 percent of faculty provided support for a student in psychological distress, yet at the same time, many respondents found it challenging and stressful to provide this sort of support to students.[41]

Providing training in this area may improve confidence and comfortability. Unfortunately, 71.4 percent of faculty in the study never attended any form of mental health training on campus. Additionally, 64 percent of respondents would welcome training in this area, and 54.9 percent of faculty reported mental health training would help them do their job.

A brief survey was administered to 14,584 faculty and staff members and 51,294 students at colleges and universities by Kognito between 2012 and 2017.[42] This brief survey was offered prior to a respondent's participation in a training course related to mental health. It is not articulated in the report, but some of the respondents may be from a community college or two-year institution.

The results indicated that, generally, faculty lack confidence and comfort around supporting students in distress, yet a strong majority (87%) believe is it their role to connect students in distress with resources. First, more than 50 percent of respondents did not feel adequately ready to recognize when a student is showing signs of psychological distress (depression, anxiety, suicide ideation). Second, more than 60 percent of respondents did not feel ready to approach a student in distress with their concern. And, finally, at least 50 percent of respondents did not feel comfortable recommending services to students in distress.

Kalkbrenner et al. conducted a phenomenological study at a midsized public four-year institution.[43] The study was focused on faculty who *actively supported* their students' mental health. In other words, the 10 participants in this study were both confident and comfortable working with students navigating mental health issues. The authors crafted five themes; some had subthemes.

The first was knowledge of mental health disorder definition(s); most saw mental health disorders (MHDs) as deriving from genetic and environmental factors. Second was knowledge of warning signs. Third was willingness to recognize and refer. All participants were accepting of students with MHDs and comfortable with referral. Fourth was limited knowledge about resources for mental health issues. Participants knew little more than the fact that a counseling center existed on campus. There was no centralized faculty resource. A lack of unity and support from university leaders were noted. Fifth, the primacy of the faculty-student relationship was highlighted.

## Influencing Factors

Several factors seem to be related to faculty actions regarding student mental health. First, faculty gender is a factor. There were some gender differences apparent within Backels and Wheeler's study.[44] Women were more likely to give flexibility for depression and test anxiety. Women were also more likely to refer for the following issues: death of a parent, family problems, eating disorders, and depression.

Faculty gender also made a difference in Becker et al.'s study.[45] Women faculty were more likely than men faculty to see themselves as able to discuss concerns with students who may have mental illness, encourage and convince students to seek help at the university counseling center, and encourage and convince students to seek help off-campus.

In more recent work, Kalkbrenner and Carlisle tested the utility of the REDFLAGS model (fully explained later in the book) to facilitate the referral of students to the counseling center by faculty.[46] Data were collected using a survey administered to faculty at a public university in the mid-Atlantic. There were 227 respondents. Overall, "increases in participants' recognition of the items on the REDFLAGS Model as warning signs for mental distress were associated with a considerable increase in the odds of having made a student referral to the counseling center."[47]

In terms of gender, male faculty members who had never been to counseling were less likely to recognize the items presented through the REDFLAGS model than female faculty members who had never been to counseling. Also, females were more aware of the warning signs within the REDFLAGS model than males.[48]

Ketchen Lipson, Talaski, and Cesare, in other recent work, found that faculty outreach efforts to students with mental health concerns vary significantly based on gender.[49] A striking 85 percent of women and 84 percent of transgender, nonbinary, genderqueer, and gender nonconforming faculty reported having these conversations versus men at 70 percent.

Second, number of years teaching, or teaching experience, is also a factor. For example, the community college faculty with more experience in Backels and Wheeler's study expressed that boyfriend or girlfriend issues had more effect; they were also more likely to refer for stress.[50]

Third, where and how information about mental health and psychiatric disabilities (PDs) is obtained matters. Brockelman et al. sought to understand the relationship between sources of information (like the media, professional training, personal relationships, and personal experiences) and faculty perceptions of working with students with PDs.[51] The authors found that faculty who reported having a friend or student with a PD or who were currently being treated for a PD tended to also have more positive perceptions of students with PDs.

Fourth, as mentioned above, personal experiences with mental health issues influence how faculty support students who may be navigating a mental health concern. More recently, Kalkbrenner et al. found that faculty with personal experiences with mental health concerns can empathize with and relate to students who may be struggling with their mental health.[52] In addition, having a positive relationship with a student was a facilitator of referral to resources. Lastly, Kalkbrenner and Carlisle found that faculty who had been to counseling were more likely to be aware of certain mental health warning signs than those who had never been to counseling.[53]

## Recommendations

Generally, Backels and Wheeler found that faculty members may not grasp
the importance of extending flexibility for and making referrals about problems that do not appear to be a crisis.[54] Advocacy for students is necessary.
Taking part in national screening surveys would be a good starting point for
campuses, they argued. Student affairs personnel and counseling center staff
ought to consider ways to educate faculty on how mental health concerns
affect students' academic performance and the importance of flexibility
and referral.

Four recommendations were derived from Kalkbrenner et al.'s study
involving faculty.[55] First, institutions should increase awareness and knowledge of the campus counseling center among faculty. Second, campus
resources and policies should be unified. Third, the academic environment
should be structured to be conducive of strong faculty-student relationships.
Fourth, institutions should advocate for college counseling centers.

Several implications were elucidated from the results of Kalkbrenner and
Carlisle's study, some of which may be helpful to community colleges.[56]
They determined that the REDFLAGS Model can be a helpful tool in training faculty to be(come) referral agents on campus. Also, faculty should be
encouraged to go to counseling because this can build empathy. Information
and resources should be provided. Lastly, they suggest encouraging men to
become aware of the warning signs of mental distress and focusing on men
with regards to educational programming.


## SUMMARY

This chapter was meant to provide an overview of the faculty and their
students within the nation's community colleges. With a few notable exceptions, community college faculty have not received much significant attention
within the literature.[57] This is a problem, as faculty are vital to the sector's
academic mission.

Understanding community college faculty members' work context; demography; preparation and professional development; work conditions; employment status; and experiences and impact is an important part of understanding
their perspectives on and experiences with their students' mental health.
Information about community college students and the community college
sector was also threaded through this section.

Because the main role of the community college faculty member is as
teacher, they touch the lives of many students. As such, their pedagogical work—and its effects on student success—is a vital, yet understudied,

component of their professional lives and their students' educational lives.[58] Until now, faculty perceptions of and experiences with community colleges student mental health were absent from the literature. Theirs is, perhaps, the best vantage point on campus relevant to this issue. Through this book, their voices will be amplified.

## NOTES

1. Frances K. Stage and Steven Hubbard, "Teaching Latino, African American, and Native American Undergraduates: Faculty Attitudes, Conditions, and Practices," in *Understanding Minority-Serving Institutions,* eds. Marybeth Gasman, Benjamin Baez, and Caroline Sotello Viernes Turner (Albany, NY: State University of New York Press, 2007), 252.

2. Patrick Sullivan, *Economic Inequality, Neoliberalism, and the American Community College* (London: Palgrave Macmillan, 2007), 149.

3. American Association of Community Colleges (AACC), "Fast Facts 2022," Research Trends, revised May 11, 2022, https://www.aacc.nche.edu/research-trends /fast-facts/.

4. The Chronicle of Higher Education, *The Almanac of Higher Education* (Washington, DC: 2022).

5. Daniel Foley, Lynn Milan, and Karen Hamrick, *The Increasing Role of Community Colleges Among Bachelor's Degree Recipients: Findings from the 2019 Survey of College Graduates* (Alexandria, VA: National Center for Science and Engineering Statistics, 2022), https://ncses.nsf.gov/pubs/nsf21309/.

6. AACC, "Fast Facts 2022."

7. Thomas R. Bailey and Irina E. Averianova, *Multiple Missions of Community Colleges: Conflicting or Complementary?* (New York: Community College Research Center, Teachers College, Columbia University, October 1998), https://ccrc.tc .columbia.edu/media/k2/attachments/multiple-missions-conflicting-complementary .pdf.

8. Gail O. Merrow and Cynthia M. Heelan, *Minding the Dream: The Process and Practice of the American Community College* (Lanham, MD: Rowman & Littlefield, 2008), 257.

9. Arthur M. Cohen, Florence B. Brawer, and Carrie B. Kisker, *The American Community College*, 6th ed. (San Francisco, CA: Jossey-Bass, 2014).

10. AACC, "Fast Facts 2022."

11. AACC, "Fast Facts 2022," (terminology used by the source).

12. AACC, "Fast Facts 2022."

13. AACC, "Fast Facts 2022."

14. See, for example Katharine M. Broton and Sara Goldrick-Rab, "Going Without: An Exploration of Food and Housing Insecurity Among Undergraduates," *Educational Researcher* 47 no. 2 (March 2018): 121–133, https://doi.org/10.3102 /0013189X17741303; Katharine M. Broton, Milad Mohebali, and Mitchel D. Lingo,

"Basic Needs Insecurity and Mental Health: Community College Students' Dual Challenges and Uses of Social Support," *Community College Review* 50 no. 4 (October 2022): 456–482, https://doi.org/10.1177/00915521221111460; J. Luke Wood and Frank Harris III, "Experiences With 'Acute' Food Insecurity Among College Students," *Educational Researcher* 47 no. 2 (March 2018): 142–145, https://doi.org/10.3102/0013189X17752928.

15. The Hope Center for College, Community, and Justice, "*#RealCollege 2021: Basic Needs Insecurity During the Ongoing Pandemic*" (Philadelphia, PA: Temple University, March 2021), https://hope.temple.edu/sites/hope/files/media/document/HopeNationalReport2021-22-compressed-compressed.pdf.

16. Broton et al., "Basic Needs Insecurity."

17. National Center for Education Statistics, "Table 315.10. Number of Faculty in Degree-Granting Postsecondary Institutions, By Employment Status, Sex, Control, and Level of Institution: Selected Years, Fall 1970 Through Fall 2020," *2020 Digest of Educational Statistics* (table prepared November 2021), https://nces.ed.gov/programs/digest/d21/tables/dt21_315.10.asp.

18. Cohen et al., *The American Community College.*

19. Cohen et al., *The American Community College*; Steven Hurlburt and Michael McGarrah, *The Shifting Academic Workforce: Where are the Contingent Faculty?* (Arlington, VA: Delta Cost Project, American Institutes for Research, 2016), https://www.air.org/resource/brief/shifting-academic-workforce-where-are-contingent-faculty.

20. See, for example, George Bulman and Robert W. Fairlie, "The Impact of COVID-19 on Community College Enrollment and Student Success: Evidence from California Administrative Data," (Working Paper 28715, National Bureau of Economic Research, Cambridge, MA, April 2021, Revised March 2022), https://doi.org/10.3386/w28715.

21. Ann E. Austin, "Preparing the Next Generation of Faculty: Graduate School as Socialization to the Academic Career," *Journal of Higher Education* 73 no. 1 (January/February 2002): 94–122, https://doi.org/10.1080/00221546.2002.11777132.

22. Kevin Kelly, "COVID-19 Planning for Fall 2020: A Closer Look at Hybrid-Flexible Course Design," *Phil on EdTech* (blog), May 7, 2020, https://philonedtech.com/covid-19-planning-for-fall-2020-a-closer-look-at-hybrid-flexible-course-design/.

23. AACC, "Fast Facts 2022."

24. Rebecca D. Cox, *The College Fear Factor: How Students and Professors Misunderstand One Another* (Cambridge, MA: Harvard University Press, 2011).

25. See Janice Nahra Friedel et al., eds., *Fifty State Systems of Community Colleges: Mission, Governance, Funding, & Accountability,* 4th ed. (Johnson City, TN: Overmountain Press, 2014).

26. National Center for Educational Statistics, "Employees and Instructional Staff: What is the Adjusted 9-Month Average Salary of Full-Time Instructional Staff Not in Medical Schools at Title IV Degree-Granting Institutions?" Trend Generator, IPEDS (Human Resources Component Final Data Fall 2016–2019 and Provisional Data Fall

2020), https://nces.ed.gov/ipeds/TrendGenerator/app/answer/5/50?f=5%3D2%3B57%3D4%7C3%3B4%3D1%7C2.

27. American Federation of Teachers, *An Army of Temps: AFT 2020 Adjunct Faculty Quality of Work/Life Report* (Washington, DC: American Federation of Teachers, AFL-CIO, 2020), https://www.aft.org/sites/default/files/media/2020/adjuncts_qualityworklife2020.pdf.

28. Judith M. Gappa, and David W. Leslie, *The Invisible Faculty: Improving the Status of Part-Timers in Higher Education* (San Francisco, CA: Wiley, 1993).

29. Carol A. Lundberg, "Peers and Faculty as Predictors of Learning for Community College Students," *Community College Review* 42 no. 2 (April 2014): 79–98, https://doi.org/10.1177/0091552113517931.

30. Lundberg, "Peers and Faculty as Predictors," 90.

31. Lauren Schudde, "Short- and Long-Term Impacts of Engagement Experiences with Faculty and Peers at Community Colleges," *Review of Higher Education* 42 no. 2 (Winter 2019): 408, https://doi.org/10.1353/rhe.2019.0001.

32. Schudde, "Short- and Long-Term Impacts," 405.

33. Natalie A. Kistner and Carrie E. Henderson, "The Drop Rate Improvement Program at Odessa College," *Achieving the Dream's Technology Solutions: Case Study Series* (Silver Spring, MD: Achieving the Dream, April 2022), https://achievingthedream.org/wp-content/uploads/2022/04/Drop-Rate-Improvement-Program-Odessa-College.pdf.

34. Kistner and Henderson, "Drop Rate Improvement Program."

35. Sarah Ketchen Lipson, Amber Talaski, and Nina Cesare, *The Role of Faculty in Student Mental Health* (Lexington, MA: Mary Christie Institute, April 2021), https://marychristieinstitute.org/wp-content/uploads/2021/04/The-Role-of-Faculty-in-Student-Mental-Health.pdf.

36. Kelsey Backels and Inese Wheeler, "Faculty Perceptions of Mental Health Issues Among College Students," *Journal of College Student Development* 42 no. 2 (2001): 173.

37. Backels and Wheeler, "Faculty Perceptions of Mental Health," 173–176.

38. Backels and Wheeler, "Faculty Perceptions of Mental Health."

39. Marion Becker et al., "Students with Mental Illnesses in a University Setting: Faculty and Student Attitudes, Beliefs, Knowledge, and Experiences," *Psychiatric Rehabilitation Journal* 25 no. 4 (Spring 2002): 359–368, https://doi.org/10.1037/h0095001.

40. Becker et al., "Students with Mental Illnesses."

41. K. L. Margrove, M. Gustowska, M., and L. S. Grove, "Provision of Support for Psychological Distress by University Staff, and Receptiveness To Mental Health Training," *Journal of Further and Higher Education* 38 no. 1 (2014): 90–106, https://doi.org/10.1080/0309877X.2012.699518.

42. Glenn Albright and Victor Schwartz, *Are Campuses Ready to Support Students in Distress? A Survey of 65,177 Faculty, Staff, and Students in 100+ Colleges and Universities* (New York: The Jed Foundation and Kognito, 2017), http://go.kognito.com/rs/143-HCJ-270/images/HiEd_WP_080817_HigherEdSurveyWhitePaper.pdf.

43. Michael T. Kalkbrenner, Amber L. Jolley, and Danica G. Hays, "Faculty Views on College Student Mental Health: Implications for Retention and Student Success," *Journal of College Student Retention: Research, Theory & Practice* 23 no. 3 (November 2021): 636–658, https://www.doi.org/10.1177/1521025119867639.

44. Backels and Wheeler, "Faculty Perceptions of Mental Health."

45. Becker et al., "Students with Mental Illnesses."

46. Michael T. Kalkbrenner and Kristie L. Carlisle, "Faculty Members and College Counseling: Utility of the REDFLAGS Model. *Journal of College Student Psychotherapy* 35 no. 1 (2021), 70–86, https://doi.org/10.1080/87568225.2019.1621230; Michael T. Kalkbrenner, "Recognizing and Supporting Students with Mental Health Disorders: The REDFLAGS Model," *Journal of Education and Training* 3 no. 1 (February 2016), http://dx.doi.org/10.5296/jet.v3i1.8141.

47. Kalkbrenner and Carlisle, "Utility of the REDFLAGS Model," 80.

48. Kalkbrenner and Carlisle, "Utility of the REDFLAGS Model."

49. Ketchun Lipson et al., *The Role of Faculty.*

50. Backels and Wheeler, "Faculty Perceptions of Mental Health."

51. Karin F. Brockelman, Janis G. Chadsey, and Jane W. Loeb, "Faculty Perceptions of University Students with Psychiatric Disabilities," *Psychiatric Rehabilitation Journal* 30 no. 1 (Summer 2006): 23–30, https://doi.org/10.2975/30.2006.23.30.

52. Kalkbrenner et al., "Faculty Views on College Student Mental Health."

53. Kalkbrenner and Carlisle, "Utility of the REDFLAGS Model."

54. Backels and Wheeler, "Faculty Perceptions of Mental Health."

55. Kalkbrenner et al., "Faculty Views on College Student Mental Health."

56. Kalkbrenner and Carlisle, "Utility of the REDFLAGS Model."

57. See, for example, Cox, *The College Fear Factor;* W. Norton Grubb and Associates, *Honored but Invisible: An Inside Look at Teaching in Community Colleges* (New York: Routledge, 1999); John S. Levin, Susan Kater, and Richard L. Wagoner, *Community College Faculty: At Work in the New Economy* (New York: Palgrave Macmillan, 2006); Greg Sethares, *The Impacts of Neoliberalism on US Community Colleges: Reclaiming Faculty Voice in Faculty Governance* (New York: Routledge, 2020).

58. Susan Twombly and Barbara K. Townsend, "Community College Faculty: What We Know and Need to Know," *Community College Review* 36 no. 1 (July 2008): 5–24, https://doi.org/10.1177/0091552108319538.

# Chapter 3

# Research on Community College Student Mental Health

"I had a student. He was *there*. He was *all* excited the first day of class. I think he came to the second one [class], and then he disappeared, and then I got an email from him. I think he was a vet, and he has bipolar disorder. And he said 'I'm in the hospital right now. I want to stay in your class. I'm real excited about it.' And I didn't see him again, and he withdrew so I know, *I know* that mental health is an issue for a number of our students."

–Eve

"But I mean, it's shocking how almost every [first-year seminar] student will write about depression and anxiety. Almost. Every. Student. [emphasis on each individual word]."

–Sophie

The research on college student mental health is well-established within the four-year institution space; far less is known about the community college sector. The literature on college student mental health rarely includes community college students, yet community college students comprise 39 percent of all undergraduate students in the United States.[1] This lack of attention has further marginalized community college students; they are a student population warranting consideration, study, and resources.[2]

Compared to research done at four-year institutions, we simply do not know enough about the mental health of community college students. However, what is known about community college student mental health paints a challenging picture. These students face more and more severe mental health issues and less access to fewer resources. Stress, anxiety, and depression are the most common issues. The prevalence of mental health issues among community college students is higher than the four-year sector, and access to mental health resources is less. The students with the most need have the least access to resources.[3]

This is a difficult situation because mental health is related to student success outcomes such as grade point average, persistence, and completion. As such, community college student mental health has been positioned as a priority for many community college campuses across the United States.

The COVID-19 pandemic, ongoing racial injustice, and a fraught political landscape have exacerbated the issue. And while the literature on community college student mental health is sparse, the issue is growing and gaining the attention of leaders and policy makers. In fact, students' mental health was the *most frequently* selected pressing issue among community college presidents in September of 2021, according to a recent survey.[4] Nearly three-quarters (73%) of public two-year college presidents surveyed selected this item.

## GROWING INTEREST IN COMMUNITY COLLEGE STUDENT MENTAL HEALTH

While some research on this topic was published in the 1990s, 2000s, and early 2010s, the literature on and attention given to community college mental health began to take off in the mid-2010s. This may have been in response to the deadly shooting at Umpqua Community College (UCC) near Roseberg, Oregon, which took place on October 1, 2015. During that morning, UCC student Chris Harper-Mercer entered his writing class and fatally shot his professor along with eight fellow students. He later died by suicide after exchanging fire with law enforcement officials.

There had been other incidents of violence at community colleges, such as a stabbing at Lone Star College in Cy Fair, Texas, in 2013 and a shooting spree in Tucson, Arizona, in 2011, committed by Jared Lee Loughner, who had been suspended from Pima Community College prior to the incident. However, the violence at UCC may have been a tipping point. That incident made national news and accelerated conversations about safety on community college campuses. Suddenly, community colleges were not immune to the scale of violence seen, for example, in 2007 at Virginia Tech, where 32 people were killed by gunfire and 17 others were wounded.

On the heels of these violent incidents was a renewed commitment among community college campus leaders to put in place enhanced safety measures. Examples include the inception of crisis management teams, protocols, and training. Behavioral intervention teams (BIT) and reporting processes were created. Increased security on campus became important. Panic button technologies (physical buttons in campus buildings, apps on mobile devices) were integrated. On-campus counseling and counseling centers became available. And an increased interest in understanding community college students' mental health was evident.

Before continuing, however, it is critical to note that conflating mental health issues or illness and violence is not accurate, helpful, or productive. As will soon be articulated, mental health concerns among community college students are widespread. Yet the proportion of those with mental health concerns who commit violent acts is miniscule. A focus on violence when considering this topic muddles the reality that many, many community college students struggle with mental health.

## WHAT WE KNOW

In what follows, the extant research on community college student mental health is highlighted and organized by topic. With a few exceptions, this chapter is focused on research specifically set within the community college.

The following sections comprise the remainder of this chapter: prevalence of mental health concerns, illnesses, or disorders; as compared to the four-year sector; mental health correlates and sources of stress and mental health concerns; student subpopulations; community colleges counseling centers, counseling, and counselors; faculty and other referral agents; students' use of resources and coping strategies; and evaluations of campus actions or interventions.

Before continuing into the subsections outlined above, however, Kasey Edwardson's work warrants attention. In 2020, Edwardson provided a bird's-eye view of the quantitative research conducted on community college student health and "a synthesis of the current health topics studied in community colleges" by reviewing 28 journal articles.[5] Unsurprisingly, one common theme was that most college student health research is done within the context of four-year institutions. And just six of the 28 articles reviewed were *focused* on mental health.

There were five take-aways. First, the research is focused on four-year institutions, not community colleges. Second, prevalence of mental health disorders is likely higher in the community college. Third, community colleges do not offer much in the way of mental health support for students. Fourth, increased awareness among community college personnel is important. Fifth, information dissemination and connecting students to services is important.

In most of the studies Edwardson reviewed, the authors deployed questionnaires specific to the study, but some used pre-existing surveys, questionnaires, and/or datasets.[6] More information about how institutions can leverage existing instruments and partner with organizations that routinely do campus mental health screenings is included in the last two chapters of this book.

## Prevalence of Mental Health Concerns, Illnesses, or Disorders

Community college students experience more and more severe mental health concerns, illnesses, or disorders than their counterparts at four-year institutions. Several studies have been conducted to assess the prevalence of mental health concerns, illnesses, or disorders among community college students.

According to Daniel Eisenberg and colleagues, approximately 50 percent of community college students are experiencing mental health issues or recently experienced a mental health issue, and only half of those students are receiving services.[7] In addition, a larger proportion of community college students experience mental health issues than their counterparts at four-year institutions.

Eisenberg et al. sent a survey to 10 community colleges across the United States and received over 4,000 responses from students.[8] They noted: "poor mental health conditions are prevalent and inadequately addressed among community college students, both in absolute terms and in comparison to students at four-year colleges and universities."[9] Depression (36%) and anxiety (29%) were the most common conditions. To compound this, community college students are less likely to access services related to mental health and fewer on-campus resources are available to them.

Sarah Ketchen Lipson and colleagues conducted the *largest* study known to report on community college student mental health prevalence and treatment.[10] Findings indicated that "prevalence of mental health problems was similar in the community college and 4-year samples, with *more than half* of students meeting criteria for one or more mental health problem(s), roughly one third screening positive for depression and anxiety, and approximately 15% reporting suicidal ideation."[11]

In addition, "community college students ages 18–22 years were more likely to screen positive for depression . . . and anxiety . . . and were more likely to report suicidal ideation" when compared to their same-aged peers within the four-year sector.[12] Within the community college sample, 56.6 percent of women and 73.9 percent of those in the LGBTQ+ community had mental health problems. Lastly, financial stress was associated with a higher prevalence of mental health problems within the total sample.

Ketchen Lipson et al. explained that "[f]urther examination of the mental health of community college students is necessary to quantify the magnitude of symptom prevalence and service use in this diverse population [of students]."[13] Data came from the Healthy Minds Study (HMS). The authors said "the current study is the first analysis of national HMS data to focus on the full population of community college students and to make comparisons with a sample of 4-year students."[14]

Ketchen Lipson et al. also noted that mental health is not often cited as a factor related to student persistence, though it is known that mental health concerns adversely affect academic outcomes.[15] It is widely accepted, however, that four-year college students perform better academically when they are in good health, which includes mental health. Yet little is known about this topic within the community college sector.

And it cannot necessarily be assumed the same holds for community college students because the student populations are different. As Edwardson has noted, extant research "has not taken a direct look at the relationship between community college student health and academic outcomes."[16] Again, this includes mental health. To be sure, academic success and student mental health are assumed to be related, but in the community college context, empirical research is lacking on this topic. This signals an important area for future inquiry.

Even though only just over five percent of the data used within Oswalt et al.'s study was from community college students, their results merit inclusion here.[17] The authors examined ACHA-ACHA II data from 2009 to 2015 (*n*=454,029), but trans students, students over the age of 25, and nondegree seeking students were, unfortunately, removed from the dataset. Self-reported mental health condition diagnoses increased during this timeframe.

Over the years there were significant increases in diagnosis and treatment for anxiety, ADHD, depression, insomnia, Obsessive-Compulsive Disorder, and panic attacks.[18] There were no significant increases in the diagnoses of the following: bipolar disorder, bulimia, and schizophrenia.[19] The authors suggested institutions "identify [mental health] as a community problem that is shared by all members of the institution."[20] This is especially timely considering the pandemic and ongoing campus concerns about student mental health.

Jennifer M. Cadigan, Jennifer C. Duckworth, and Christine M. Lee examined the self-reported health needs of community college students attending institutions in the Pacific Northwest.[21] The administered survey was part of a screening tool for a larger study. The instrument included four measures: demographic characteristics, alcohol and marijuana use, mental and physical health, and health issues.

One of the items within the instrument asked participants to "List three health issues facing Community College students today."[22] Sixty percent of the respondents listed a mental health issue. Of all 2,656 issues listed, approximately 36 percent were medical and approximately 33 percent were mental. The most common mental health issues listed were stress and depression.

Once data were disaggregated, some interesting patterns emerged.[23] Women were more likely to list a mental health issue than men. Students between the ages of 18 and 29 were more likely to list two or three mental health issues as compared to older students. The authors asserted that "[p]rogrammatic efforts to support community college students and promote prevention/interventions for depression, stress reduction strategies, improving sleep, in addition to general medical concerns, remain essential."[24]

## As Compared to Four-Year Institutions

While it is interesting to compare student mental health across sectors of higher education, contexts are unique and sometimes completely indiscernible from one another. For sundry reasons, using research conducted within the four-year institution sector to inform practice at the community college level is problematic. The students, contexts, missions, and purposes of these two sectors of higher education are very different. The literature overviewed below draws comparisons between the sectors.

Daniel Seth Katz and Karen Davison used data from the spring 2010 administration of the American College Health Association–National College Health Assessment II (ACHA-NCHA II) to conduct a comparative analysis of mental health between community college students and students enrolled at four-year institutions in California.[25] The researchers found several statistically significant mental health–related differences between the two groups: "community college students [have] more severe psychological concerns and fewer institutional resources than traditional university students."[26]

The authors suggested that these differences might be attributable to differences "between student demographics, cultural issues, and motives for attending community colleges."[27] The major implication of this study was that community colleges must build infrastructure for comprehensive mental health resources—for both students and faculty and staff. Students need access to care, and faculty and staff need access to information about students' mental health needs.

Monica L. Heller and Jerrell C. Cassady's study provided some evidence of how theories considered axiomatic in the four-year realm do not translate well into the community college setting.[28] They were interested in understanding which factors predict student success based on the triadic reciprocal model.

The model (based on Albert Bandura's work) includes three factors: environmental (institution type), behavioral (self-regulated learning strategies), and personal (motivation and academic anxiety).[29] Student success was measured by GPA. Respondents were from a four-year institution and a community college. The model worked for university students but not for community college students.

About this, Heller and Cassady said "the large body of research on student success in college gathered in traditional university settings may have little bearing on supporting community college students."[30] Also, the measures were built based on students at four-year institutions. They also noted "[t]he data illustrate that the models for explaining likely student success that are based on traditional university students do not translate well to a community college population drawn from the same geographic area."[31]

Heller and Cassady noted that Bronfenbrenner's ecological model may be more appropriate for understanding student success within the two contexts, and this possibility will be addressed in later chapters of this book.[32] The authors also said "[t]he data indicate that for the community college student, the social context and educational environment become most influential to their academic success."[33]

Attrition among community college students typically has little to do with academic ability or potential; it has everything to do with circumstances beyond the college classroom. Heller and Cassady's study, among others, provides evidence for why caution must be used when applying knowledge created within the four-year context to other sectors of higher education.[34]

## Mental Health Correlates

This section is about mental health correlates. Mental health correlates are things that have been shown to have a relationship with mental health. Examples include race, gender, financial situation, and stress. This section contains three subsections: interpersonal violence (IPV), sexual violence, and stress.

While Daniel Eisenberg, Justin Hunt, and Nicole Speer's study was not focused on community college students, and it is unclear whether community colleges were included in the sample, their work merits inclusion here.[35] They argued much is known about the general picture of mental health concerns among college students (within four-year institutions) but do not have a good picture of mental health correlates.

Understanding the correlates may help institutional personnel incorporate mental health resources into the college experience more effectively. Within their study, the following correlates were examined: "demographic characteristics, academic level, religiosity, relationship status, sexual orientation, and financial situation."[36]

Data came from the Health Minds Study between fall 2007 and spring 2009. The sample included graduate and undergraduate students. There was no reference to community colleges. Nearly one third (32%) of respondents had at least one of the following mental health issues: depression, anxiety disorder, and suicide ideation. Fifteen percent of the sample engaged in non-suicidal self-harm such as cutting or punching objects.

Several additional relevant findings were reported. For example, women experienced anxiety significantly more than men. Minoritized racial groups experienced depression more than white people. Living on campus was related to being less anxious. Being very religious was related to having fewer mental health concerns. Being in a relationship meant less mental health problems. Gay, lesbian, and bisexual students were more likely to be at risk for mental health problems. Finally, past and current financial struggles were related to elevated risk for mental health problems. This last finding is highly relevant to this book, as will become clear later.

## Interpersonal Violence (IPV)

Prior to Rachel J. Voth Schrag and Tonya E. Edmond's work, no previous study examined the impact of interpersonal violence (IPV) on community college students.[37] The researchers administered a survey to a random sample of community college students across several community colleges. They sought "to describe exposure to IPV, sexual assault, and other types of trauma, as well as the burden of PTSD symptomology [sic], among female students attending . . . community colleges."[38]

Results indicated 27 percent of women community college students experienced intimate partner violence within the past 12 months; this is significantly higher than in the general population and the female undergraduate population who reported ever having a partner. This is concerning because, as the authors state, female community college students "may be facing an increase in risk of violence due to their choice to pursue power through education."[39]

Social exchange theory as a theoretical frame illustrates how (a) earning a credential changes the power dynamics within a relationship and (b) earning a credential could help a woman leave an abusive partner.[40] Therefore, abusive partners may attempt to keep women community college students from earning a credential, and this is likely to be *much* more prevalent among community college students as compared to students at four-year institutions because of the differences in the two populations.

Also, more than half (56%) of women community college students reported experiencing at least one type of trauma in their lifetimes.[41] Nearly 20 percent of women community college students have PTSD *currently*. That is one in five women community college students, which is significant.

Voth Schrag and Edmond's work "provides clear evidence that community college students are experiencing violence and the accompanying mental health impacts."[42] They noted that "[w]hen working to develop academic safety plans with survivors, advocates and counselors in the community college setting should consider the ongoing impact of trauma on learning and memory, [and] developing strategies to support survivors."[43]

Brief trauma interventions were also suggested.[44] In addition, the authors advocate for locating, deploying, and contextualizing evidence-based treatments to enhance the safety of survivors. A coordinated response across the college and community could help keep survivors safe and help them achieve their academic and personal goals as well.[45]

## Sexual Violence

Little is known about sexual violence victimization among community college students. Clery Act data only tells one part of the story. So much goes unreported (90%), and much of what happens to community college students happens off-campus with nonstudents as perpetrators. At the same time, there is a large body of literature on this topic in the context of four-year institution students.

Data used in Rebecca M. Howard et al.'s study came from a campus climate survey administered within seven community colleges in a single northeastern state.[46] The authors looked at the relationship between sexual violence victimization and well-being, which includes academic engagement, mental health, and life satisfaction. The instrument used was the Administrator Researcher Campus Climate Collaborative (ARC3) Climate Survey. White students and women students were overrepresented in the sample.

Almost half of the participants (48.4%) in the study experienced some form of sexual violence victimization while a community college student.[47] Women (51.1% reported victimization) and transgender or nonbinary students (73.1% reported victimization) were more likely to experience sexual violence victimization than men (38.8% reported victimization).

In addition, participants of color were more likely to experience sexual violence victimization than white participants.[48] Nonheterosexual students were more likely to experience sexual violence victimization than heterosexual students. Students under the age of 25 were more likely to experience sexual violence victimization than those 26 or older. Participants living with a partner and/or children were less likely to experience sexual violence victimization than those living in other kinds of living arrangements.

Furthermore, participants who experienced victimization had significantly lower mental health scores.[49] Polyvictimization (i.e., when someone experiences multiple types of victimization, such as physical abuse, sexual abuse, emotional abuse, bullying) has very negative effects on well-being. These findings are consistent with the literature on sexual violence victimization at four-year institutions. Prevalence is high and highly problematic. Howard and colleagues recommended assessment, collaboration with community agencies, adapting programming for the student population, and finding ways to share information with online students.[50]

## Stress

When stress is experienced routinely and unceasingly, mental health can suffer. In other words, the more often someone experiences stress, the more likely their mental health is to be poor. Emily A. Pierceall and Maybelle C. Keim were interested in the degree of stress perceived by community college students.[51] Approximately 13 percent of respondents reported low stress, 75 percent reported moderate stress, and 12 percent reported high stress.

Several additional results were shared.[52] There was no significant difference in perceived stress between younger (18–23) students and older students (24+). In general, women perceived more stress than men. There was no significant difference in perceived stress based on enrollment density, program type, GPA, or plans to transfer. However, students least confident in their educational goals were more stressed.

The most common ways to cope with stress among the sample were talk to family and friends (77%), leisure activities (57%), exercise (51%), drink alcohol (39%), and smoke (37%). Only 5 percent talked with a professional to cope. Unsurprisingly, students interested in a stress reduction workshop perceived more stress than those who were not interested.

Four recommendations were articulated by Peirceall and Keim.[53] First, information about personal and academic stress should be shared with students. Second, stress reduction should be added to extant wellness education efforts. Third, personnel should be informed about students' stress. Finally, community colleges ought to regularly assess students' stress levels. Again, this will be addressed later in the book.

## Student Subpopulations

Because the community college student population is so diverse, many scholars have highlighted mental health differences among students, based on the students' socio-demographic characteristics. Gender and age are examples. Furthermore, some scholars have opted to focus their inquiries on specific student subgroups. Some of these student subpopulations include student veterans, students of color, students who drink heavily, rural and urban students, single-parenting students, student-athletes, and students with adverse childhood experiences (ACEs).

## Differences Related to Gender

While there was no mention of trans or nonbinary participants, which signals a need within future research, Paris Scott Strom and colleagues found several differences between men and women.[54] Ongoing research on this topic must consider a full spectrum of gender identity beyond the narrow and exclusive man-woman binary. Trans and nonbinary students must be included in inquiries going forward so a fuller picture of differences related to gender is possible.

Notwithstanding the above commentary, differences related to gender were as follows.[55] Women experienced more stress in getting along with family members. Women also hoped family members would lower their expectations. Relatedly, women wished friends would not pressure them to answer text messages and wanted more uninterrupted study time. Women were also more likely to notice stress based on headaches or stomach aches and likely to worry about paying for college. Women were more likely to handle stress by sleeping. Finally, women were more optimistic about the potential benefits of a stress workshop at the college.

On the other hand, men were more likely to handle stress by doing physical activity or playing video games.[56] Men were also more likely to recover from losing a competition. And, lastly, men were more optimistic about their futures.

There were some additional results connected to stress but not significantly different based on gender, which Strom et al. framed as implications of the study.[57] They are as follows: time management is important, living with parents can be a stressor, peer support is an asset, instructor encouragement and support is valued, career awareness and exploration is important, understanding labor market forecasts is important, and managing the cost of college is important.

## Differences Related to Age

Laura Martin and Lynn Bohecker were interested in age-based differences.[58] They compared anxiety, depression, positive coping, and negative coping among three different age groups of community college students: 18–28, 29–39, and 40–67. There were 812 participants.

There were differences in both anxiety and depression. With regards to anxiety, the oldest group (40–67) experienced the least anxiety in terms of their median score, and there was a significant difference between the youngest (18–28) and oldest groups. In terms of depression, when the two older groups were combined, there was a significant difference between that group and the younger group. The youngest group had significantly higher depression scores.

There were also differences related to coping. The oldest group had statistically higher positive coping than the younger two groups. Younger students engaged in negative coping more than the two older groups. Overall, the youngest group experienced more anxiety and depression. The youngest group also engaged in more negative coping than the two older groups.

Based on these results, Martin and Bohecker offered several implications.[59] These included teaching positive coping skills; targeting interventions based on age; deploying telehealth, engaging faculty and staff in professional development; disaggregating student mental data by academic area, which would be helpful for faculty understandings of their students; and hiring highly skilled counselors.

## Student Veterans

John C. Fortney and colleagues compared help-seeking behaviors between veteran and civilian community college students.[60] They explained that because "there is virtually no information about treatment seeking among community college students, we examined correlates of mental health service use in this population."[61] This is vital when building interventions. For example, if veterans have higher rates of mental health concerns and are less likely to seek treatment, this could become a target population.

There were several results.[62] First, a large portion of the participants screened positive for depression (32%), generalized anxiety disorder (30%), PTSD (22%), and binge drinking (36%), yet veterans were more likely to screen positive for depression and PTSD. Next, over half of participants (57%) reported perceived need for mental health treatment; 66 percent and 59 percent of respondents thought therapy and medication would be helpful, respectively.

About one third of participants were taking psychotropic medications. However, veterans were less likely to think medication would help and more likely to perceive public stigma. Also, students aged 23 and older were more likely to be taking medications compared to students aged 22 and younger. Finally, 11 percent of participants received psychotherapy in the last year. A positive PTSD screen was a predictor of therapy.

Unfortunately, results also "indicated that community college students with a probable mental disorder or perceived need for treatment had low rates of mental health service use."[63] The screening instrument(s) used did not predict for medication use. On the other hand, the authors found that "students with greater perceived need for treatment and treatment effectiveness were more likely to use psychotropic medications."[64]

Fortney et al. articulated two main conclusions: (a) "[e]ngagement interventions that focus on increasing the perceived need for and effectiveness of treatment may be helpful in encouraging younger students to seek treatment" and (b) "engagement interventions should focus on linking students with off-site services."[65]

## Students of Color

Everything about mental health must be understood within a cultural context. Meekyung Han and Helen Pong noted how in some Asian cultures mental illness is *highly* stigmatized.[66] The authors administered a pencil and paper survey to Asian American students within a single California community college. The sample consisted of 66 students.

Nearly two-thirds of respondents said they would seek help if they had mental health problems, and women were more likely to seek help. Help seeking was related to students being highly acculturated into American society, and those who indicated a willingness to seek help were more acculturated into American society. Willingness to seek help was related to low levels of mental health stigma. Negative mental health stigma negatively affected help seeking. And acculturation into American society positively affected help seeking. Finally, knowing about mental health resources also increased the likelihood of help seeking.

Shame, coupled with stigma, played a role in the results. Seeking outside help could signal going against the high importance of family and be a sign of weakness. Based on these results, Han and Pong gave several recommendations.[67]

First, more outreach is needed, to students and to outside resources. Second, ongoing training on cultural understanding is necessary across campus. Third, educational programming to destigmatize mental health should be offered, focused on Asian American students. Fourth, institutional leaders should consider whether staff racial demographics mirror the student body. Lastly, online support and online support groups for Asian American students should be made available.

It is well rehearsed in the literature that trauma leads to mental health issues. And trauma is prevalent among college students. This has implications for academic performance and student success outcomes. Jeanne L. Edman, Susan B. Watson, and David J. Patron studied a diverse, multiethnic sample of community college students and examined to what extent there was a relationship between trauma and reported measures of psychological distress.[68]

Relevant results were as follows. Black and Latinx/a/o students reported higher instances of interpersonal violence than white students. Black students exposed to interpersonal trauma were at similar risk for depression as white students. There was a relationship between interpersonal trauma and PTSD and between depression and disordered eating attitudes. There was also a relationship between interpersonal trauma and depression.[69]

While community colleges cannot control student exposure to off-campus trauma, these exposures affect students' learning and success. The following recommendations were made by Edman et al.: educate students about trauma as it relates to mental health and academic success and provide appropriate support; educate faculty about student trauma levels; increase the larger community's awareness of interpersonal trauma; and make state governments aware of the high levels of traumatic experiences among community college students.[70]

Emalinda McSpadden provided a useful and excellent piece based on an action research project with the goal of building an effective set of intervention strategies.[71] Data were collected through focus groups; thematic analysis was deployed. The purpose of the study was to better understand students' orientations to mental health—whether a negative stigma was present—and to learn about students' mental health concerns and needs. All participants were from minoritized racial-ethnic groups. The site was an urban community college in New York City categorized as an Hispanic-Serving Institution (HSI).

The results of McSpadden's study were as follows, bundled into three categories.[72] The first category was culture-bound themes specific to mental health issues and services. Help seeking for mental health needs was seen as personal weakness. Familial stigmatization was a concern. There were negative attitudes toward discussing mental health related to familial taboo and fear of negative public perception. In addition, there was a culturally specific mistrust of mental health services. Reliance on friends and faith and self-work was normalized. There was also a belief that therapy would impede personal-professional (upward) movement.

The second category included themes specific to mental health issues and services but not explicitly culturally based. There was a general mistrust of psychotherapy, perceived lack of need (relative to personal environment/history), and a preference to talk to friends. The rationale was that friends are known and familiar and can care in the way a therapist cannot.

The third category was comprised of themes specific to seeking mental health services on campus. Mistrust of the college was prevalent, and personnel were not viewed as helpful or approachable. There was discomfort with taking initiative to seek help, attributed to a lack of confidence. Students would rather be asked if help is needed. There was a general wariness about speaking to campus personnel about personal/emotional issues. Students were cautious about information being on permanent record or hurting their academic standing by voicing a need for support and services.

Additionally, students lacked awareness of available services for various reasons. Students saw this as the college's fault for not communicating well. The commuter campus context as impediment to awareness of available services. Furthermore, students did not see the college as a place to "hang out or live your life."[73] Students viewed the college environment as incongruent with mental health services. Students felt there should be a separation between the college and personal matters, especially in light of students being adults.

Several implications were provided. First, services should include education, with the purpose of lessening stigma. Second, education should be intentional and culturally relevant. Third, information should be provided to faculty regarding outreach about services, referrals, and education, Fourth, efforts should be made to debunk mental health stigma. Fifth, peer education should be leveraged.

## Students Who Drink Heavily

The sample for Jennifer M. Cadigan and Christine M. Lee's study included community college students who drink heavily.[74] The following were examined: symptoms of mental health issues; resource utilization and perception of unmet needs; and barriers to resource utilization. Data used within this article were taken from a larger study meant to "adapt a brief intervention for high-risk alcohol use with [community college] students."[75] The larger study was also meant to see if the protective behavioral strategies intervention could be done with web-conferencing and text messages.

Results of Cadigan and Lee's work were as follows. Among the respondents, 35.2 percent screened positive for depression or anxiety. While 28.4 percent reported they had received mental health services in the past 12 months, 40.8 percent reported unmet mental health services need. Barriers to mental health service utilization included: thought they could handle the issue on their own (74.1%), did not have time (48.3%), could not afford cost (37.9%), did not think treatment would help (36.2%), and did not know where to go (31.0%). Those with a mental health issue noted cost as a barrier more so, and more barriers overall, than those without.[76]

Even though the research on community college student mental health is growing, barriers to service utilization remain under-researched. That approximately 41 percent of the students in Cadigan and Lee's study had an unmet mental health services need is significant; this is a higher percentage than students at a four-year institution and young adults in general (comparable population).[77] Removing barriers to access is vital. And access to educational materials is important, as many participants thought they could handle the situation on their own.

As is consistently reported in the literature, community college students are reporting more barriers to mental health service, and they are also in the greatest need for services.[78] The authors make a financial case for increasing support for community college students' mental health. They said, "[t]raining of all student services personnel staff and faculty in evidence-based practices such as motivational interviewing and screening for mental health or substance abuse may be a worthwhile and cost-effective endeavor."[79] This will be further explicated in the final two chapters of this text.

## *Rural and Urban Students*

Urbanicity is an important factor for any community college and its student body, and this includes understanding and supporting student mental health. Stacy Waters-Bailey, Matthew S. McGraw, and Jason Barr provided strategies for building support resources for rural community college students who may be facing food and/or housing insecurity, lack of transportation and/or childcare, and unmet mental health care needs.[80] Yet customization based on individual campus needs is vital. As the authors argue, "an issue that may be paramount in one locality may barely exist or not be an issue in another."[81] The student population and local community must be taken into serious account.

Only a small portion of Waters-Bailey et al.'s piece is dedicated to mental health, yet they offered some useful suggestions.[82] First, they suggested forming partnerships to carry out assessments. Second, access to off-campus mental health resources may be particularly difficult for students living in rural areas. On-campus resources would be ideal. But rural community colleges can also provide students with information on what is available close by. To close, the authors asserted that "a community college can, with some planning and copious amounts of administrative support, reduce the nonacademic barriers that many students face."[83]

Lesley Rennis and colleagues were interested in how urban community college students access the internet for health–related information, including mental health.[84] eHealth Literacy is a version of health literacy, which is an individual's ability to seek, locate, and understand health information. Appraisal of information is important within eHealth Literacy. They concluded that "several students used the Internet in place of conventional health care services, mostly to avoid medical costs."[85]

Lack of health/medical insurance contributed to this; these students were very concerned about health care costs. Internet use among participants in this study tended to be reactive (after there is a health problem) and diagnostic (used to determine what is wrong). While this can be framed as an economically rational choice by students, eHealth Literacy skills should accompany this behavior. The authors noted that "care must be taken to give students ample opportunity to process eHealth information at a deeper level in order to develop skills in effectively evaluating personal health information found online."[86]

## Single-Parenting Students

Single-parenting students make up a significant portion of the community college student body at 15 percent.[87] This is an important student subpopulation, and community colleges must endeavor to customize services and resources to meet their needs. Divya Shenoy, Christine Lee, and Sang Leng Trieu conducted a secondary analysis of ACHA-NCHA data collected during the spring of 2013.[88]

Most of the single-parent students were female (82.2%). The most significant finding was that the rate of suicide attempts reported by single parents was double that of the rest of the sample. The authors noted that "[f]or single parents, all mental health indicators may merit increased attention; however, the higher rates of suicide ideation and attempts are particularly alarming, given that these students support children who depend on them."[89]

Single-parenting students who have many sometimes competing demands on their time and energy "may experience a higher incidence of mental health difficulties, including suicide ideation and attempts."[90] One positive note, however, was that "single-parenting students reported being more likely to seek help from professionals when faced with adverse life circumstances."[91]

## Student-Athletes

Research related to the psychological well-being of community college student-athletes is sparse, yet over 70,000 student-athletes compete within the National Junior College Athletic Association (NJCAA) annually.[92] Joshua C. Watson sought to understand the relationship between perceived stress, locus of control, and athletic identity among community college student-athletes.[93]

Being a student-athlete is stressful during an ordinarily stressful time (i.e., college).[94] Some causes of stress include extensive travel for competitions, exhausting training, and the pressure to win. Two factors or constructs thought to be related to student-athlete stress are locus of control and athletic identity.

Results were as follows. Men were less stressed and had stronger athletic identities than women. African American and Hispanic participants tended to have a more internalized locus of control than white participants. A significant positive correlation existed between stress and locus of control (external) and between stress and athletic identity. Student-athletes with an external locus of control saw themselves as having more stress. And, the more student-athletes identified as athletes, the more stress they saw in their lives.[95]

The results of this study suggest specific attention ought to be given to community college student-athletes' mental health. Student-athletes must juggle a lot and, as a result, there are a lot of demands on their time and energy. While there are benefits to being a student-athlete, there are also costs. Watson said "[t]he more students identify with the athlete role, the more invested they are in the athletic demands of their time and energy," and one cost associated with an extensive investment in their sport is potentially "neglecting other aspects of the college experience including academic pursuits."[96]

The following recommendations were provided: (a) targeting interventions; (b) ensuring access to services like academic advising and career counseling; (c) offering stress management programming; (d) providing group sessions to process stress; (e) giving transfer assistance, as this is process is stressful and most students are not successful; and (f) offering campus personnel education around the athlete identity.[97]

### Students with Adverse Childhood Experiences (ACEs)

Laura Brogden and Dennis E. Gregory aimed to understand how ACEs may affect community college students and what role resiliency may play in terms of success outcomes.[98] They studied adult community college students with three or more ACEs as they entered the postsecondary space. This was a qualitative study; the authors used interpretive phenomenological analysis. Students had completed 24 credits and filled out a "widely recognized ACE survey"[99] to determine eligibility.

Analysis yielded five themes.[100] First, most participants experienced anxiety and depression. About half had ADHD. Second, participants were unsure whether they could succeed, and expressed a lack of deservingness. There was also a lack of confidence. Third, overwhelming stress was a constant in most participants' lives. Fourth, many of the participants were still in the presence of people who caused them harm (e.g., family members). Often, the ACEs have long-lasting effects and can become generational. Lastly, despite the odds, participants continued with their educational pursuits; they were persistent.

There were several implications for practice.[101] They included: presence of mental health centers; educational programming about ACEs and stress reduction; opportunities to develop skills like goal-setting and study stills; financial support included with basic needs resources; early connection with faculty; and use of trauma-informed practices.

## Community College Counselors, Counseling, and Counseling Centers

The *community college counselor,* as a term, is a relic of the *high school counselor*, which illustrates how early community colleges were born out of the K-12 environment. Community college counselors, a term and role that still exists today, engage in work similar to school counselors, doing the work of a mental health counselor, academic advisor, and career development professional (i.e., to address the personal, academic, and career-related concerns of students).

At the same time, student affairs professionals at community colleges are often cross-trained within a number of functional areas.[102] Budget constraints, campus size, and limited students' campus presence have contributed to this.[103] The uniqueness of the community college student population must be considered as it relates to professional preparation for mental health counselors, academic advisors, and career development educators. The counselor position has undergone, and continues to undergo, significant changes as these institutions and their students evolve.

Many of the historical roles of a counselor are now broken up into specialty positions within higher education broadly because the work has become too big. This is even the case in some K-12 contexts (e.g., career and college readiness positions). However, and as mentioned above, in some community colleges, *all-purpose* counselors do still exist, and in some cases these folks are tenured or on the tenure track.

Some early research on this topic showed that the needs of community college counselors may not have been met through mental health counseling, school counseling, or college student personnel master's programs and that only some elements of these programs were relevant for community college counselors.[104] This suggested that community college counselors spent most of their time each week focused on academic advising. One study found that community college counselors spent about six hours per week providing personal counseling, above and beyond the career counseling they were also offering.[105]

Even back then, there were concerns about the lack of professional development opportunities available to community college counselors. Offering more professional development is a good start, but it also must be relevant and of high quality.[106]

Historically, the emphasis for the community college counselor position has been the academic and career needs of students, though research from as early as in the 2000s found that some of the student issues counselors may encounter included depression, stress and anxiety, and alcohol and other drug use.[107] And as is evident above, community college students' need for mental health support has risen to overwhelming levels, making it a top priority for leaders. Generally speaking, more *mental health* counseling centers and *mental health* counselors on community college campuses are desperately needed.[108]

## Community College Counseling Centers

The presence of an on-campus counseling center is ideal in addressing student mental health concerns. There are several arguments for this.[109] First, the on-campus comprehensive counseling center can support the multiple missions of the community college. Second, counseling supports academic success, retention, and transfer and graduation rates. Third, there is an increased demand; students are coming to campus with more mental health issues. Fourth, students with mental health problems can affect other students and the institution in negative ways. Fifth, counseling interventions can help with retention and attrition.

The vision put forward within Dykes-Anderson's piece was more comprehensive than just attending to students' mental health.[110] The author advocated for "holistic and comprehensive" programming that encompasses academic advising; career coaching; transfer advising; personal counseling, diagnostic screening and referrals, and crisis intervention; outreach programming, teaching (counselors should teach first-year seminar courses); faculty education; and program evaluation.[111]

While many student affairs units on community college campuses have moved toward one-stop or single-stop centers where students can access functions such as advising, financial aid, career development, and disability services, most counseling centers on community college campuses are dedicated to supporting students' wellness and mental health. The vision advocated by Dykes-Anderson has not yet been widely realized.[112]

## Faculty and Other Referral Agents

In conducting a literature search on the topic of community college student mental health, *only one* study was located that focused on the experiences of faculty. Ethan and Seidel wanted to understand how these faculty saw their role in helping students with nonacademic problems, their awareness of resources and policies related to student mental health, and recommendations for supporting other faculty.[113]

Students will often connect with their faculty about things like stress, anxiety, and other nonacademic issues before going to the campus counseling center. Because faculty are "professionals in the college community whom students see regularly and often develop trust in, college faculty are on the front lines of student crisis."[114]

Three themes were articulated. The first was faculty experiences with students in distress and their impressions about student resiliency and students' ability to manage their role sets. Ethan and Seidel said they were "witness to the delicate space between teacher and student marked by the student's trust and vulnerability and the teacher's concern beyond the parameters of the classroom."[115]

Faculty were sometimes confident in their approaches to students, but not always. The faculty "often 'sensed' something was wrong but did not know how or whether to address the matter with the student."[116] Some examples included: student clutching their backpack during class, student softly murmuring during class, and a student repeatedly sitting in the back corner.

The second theme was that while faculty were aware the counseling center existed, they were unsure of what happened there. There was a tendency for faculty to refer to people on campus they knew. Faculty reported a lack of formal training on supporting and handling students in distress. While faculty in the study were "demonstrating authentic and caring efforts toward students in distress," it was acknowledged that working "with complicated students without adequate support can rob time and emotional energy from the already demanding life of a college professor."[117]

The third theme was recommendations offered by faculty participants. These included the following: raise awareness of services; connect specific counselors to academic departments, and invite counselors to faculty meetings; curate and share information on policies, procedures, and resources related to students in distress; create protocols for after-hours situations; launch an aggressive public relations campaign regarding mental health and counseling; list counseling center information inside syllabi; provide faculty with slides to show in class or otherwise share with students; and generate posters and screen content related to wellness and mental health.

Faculty also expressed a desire for increased administrative support. They felt "like well-meaning actions could leave them vulnerable to scrutiny, perhaps placing their jobs and even their likelihood to earn tenure at risk."[118] More support for faculty related to this issue should be provided among community college leaders.

Based on these three themes, Ethan and Seidel also offered their own recommendations.[119] They are as follows: leverage web-based resources (e.g., https://kognito.com/); implement Mental Health First Aid training (see https://www.mentalhealthfirstaid.org/); empower students with various resources (in-person and online/virtual); bring mental health awareness and services into the institution's culture; encourage faculty to work alongside student affairs professionals on this issue; fold training on student mental health into new faculty orientation; and involve faculty in the behavioral intervention team.

## Referral Agents

Faculty are not the only people on campus who regularly interface with students. Students are also in contact with a variety of personnel as well as other students. Anyone with whom a student has contact on campus could serve as a referral agent. This may include student affairs staff, librarians, campus security, and students. Referral agents are those who can point students to available on- and off-campus services and/or supports.

Michael Kalkbrenner and Thomas J. Hernández analyzed archival data to understand the relationship between residential community college students' awareness of mental health disorders (MHD) and their propensity to refer a friend who presented signs of an MHD to facilitative (e.g., referral to counseling center) and debilitative resources (e.g., encourage consumption of alcohol).[120] The researchers found there was a "statistically significant main effect for awareness of MHDs and the likelihood that participants would refer a friend to facilitative resources."[121]

Participants with high levels of MHD awareness were more likely to refer a friend showing MHD signs to facilitative resources than participants with low levels of MHD awareness. In addition, males were more likely to refer friends showing MHD signs to debilitative resources. But at the same time, "female students did not report a higher willingness than male students to refer a friend who was showing signs of a MHD to facilitative resources at a statistically significant level."[122]

Based on these results, it is important for community college administrators to champion efforts to raise students' levels of awareness of the signs of MHDs among classmates as well as the importance of referral to facilitative resources. This could include syllabus statements, educational programming, and marketing and communication campaigns.

Campus referral agents must have some level of mental health literacy to refer students to appropriate resources. The REDFLAGS model is used to promote mental health literacy within higher education,[123] yet it has only recently gained traction at the community college level. The model is as follows.

- **R**ecurrent class absences that are sudden or uncharacteristic of the student
- **E**xtreme and unusual emotional reactions
- **D**ifficulty concentrating
- **F**requent display of anxiety or worry about class assignments

- Late or incomplete assignments turned in abruptly and with increasing frequency
- Apathy toward personal appearance and hygiene
- Gut feeling that something does not seem right
- Sudden deterioration in the quality of work or content of work becomes negative or dark

The model helps campus personnel with decision making about counseling referrals. Validating its use for community college students is necessary considering the needs of the students in the sector. Many of the characteristics of community college students are consistent with characteristics often connected with mental health concerns.

Mental health literacy is a newer concept. It is related to knowledge and beliefs, attitudes toward, and understandings of resources related to mental health. According to Kalkbrenner et al., "research has yet to validate the utility of a specific model of mental health literacy (e.g., the REDFLAGS model) with the community college student population."[124]

Therefore, Kalkbrenner et al. remedied that.[125] In short, the model works within the community college arena. The authors asserted that the "REDFLAGS model represents an empirically tested and unidimensional model of recognizable warning signs of mental distress in community college students."[126] Previous attendance in counseling significantly affected the respondents' scores. This was the only independent variable that affected the scores in a significant way.

The model could be an effective tool for referral training. Women, because they are more likely to refer, should be recruited as peer referral agents.[127] Also, men and nonwhite students should be targeted for mental health awareness training. The findings also suggested community college students may be accessing counseling at the same rate at students at four-year institutions. They also make peer referrals at the same frequency. Students who had attended counseling were more likely to recognize the model's items as mental health concern warning signs. Students with a help-seeking history may make good peer referral agents.

## Students' Use of Resources and Coping Strategies

Some research has been conducted on community college students' use of resources and coping strategies. Resources may include going to therapy, seeking counseling, and/or taking prescribed psychotropic medications under the guidance of a medical professional. Coping strategies are often conceived as existing on a continuum between adaptive or positive and maladaptive or negative. Examples of the former may include taking a walk, talking with a friend, or using mental health apps. Examples of the latter include avoidance or using alcohol.

## Therapy and Medication

The results of Sarah Ketchen Lipson et al.'s study indicated that "[a]mong students with one or more reported mental health problems, community college students had lower rates of therapy within the last year . . . relative to 4-year students."[128] Approximately one-third of students in the sample were using psychotropic medication, a similar proportion between community college and four-year institution students. Only 5.4 percent of community college students who used services did so on campus as compared to 23.4 percent of four-year students, yet these kinds of services are much less readily available within the community college sector.

While one-third of white students used therapy, only 6.8 percent of Arab and 18.2 percent of Latinx students used therapy. Community college students aged 18 to 22 were less likely than their same-age four-year counterparts to use treatment; they also used psychotropic medication less. And, finally, financial constraints were the most common barrier to treatment among community college students; for four-year students it was not having enough time.

## Online Mental Health Resources

Because so little is known about community college student attitudes about online mental health services, Michael S. Dunbar and colleagues conducted one of the first and largest studies focused on community college student use and perceptions of online mental health services within the United States.[129] They found that, among students with need for mental health support, less than 10 percent had ever used on-campus services exclusively, less than 30 percent had ever used on- or off-campus services, and only three percent had ever used online services exclusively. That means a staggering 70 percent of students who could have benefited from mental health services did not receive any in any format. The authors also noted that "[s]tudents with treatment need and a history of in-person treatment were more likely to prefer face-to-face treatment over online therapy, whereas students with no prior in-person treatment were less likely to prefer in-person services."[130] This finding suggests that online services may be an effective gateway to treatment for students who have never received it. Online services may also supplement in-person treatment, and this may especially be the case during a pandemic, for example. Efforts to promote online mental health services on community college campuses ought to emphasize their flexibility and convenience.

## Mental Health Apps

For community colleges to effectively deploy a mental health application for smart phones ("app," for short), research is necessary. Institutions need to understand whether students have phones, whether they use apps already, and whether there is interest. There have been some initial steps within that area.[131]

Judith Borghouts and colleagues sought to understand what factors lead to mental health app usage among community college students.[132] They examined the following factors: perception of need to help-seek for mental health issues, perception of stigma, past use of mental health services, worries about privacy, and influence of others who use mental health apps.[133]

Demographic results of the survey were as follows (survey administration was at the height of the pandemic).[134] First, nearly 40 percent of participants reported experiencing or having mental illness. Second, over 40 percent of participants reported experiencing a mental health concern from stress. Third, more than half of participants harbored a moderate to severe perceived (negative) stigma related to mental health. Fourth, over 20 percent of participants used a mental health app.

Barriers to accessing mental health resources were as follows.[135] Students preferred to deal with issues on their own; this could be related to help-seeking stigma. There were also privacy concerns. Students questioned the seriousness of their needs. Finally, students worried about what others will think of them for accessing mental health resources.

There were some important results related to mental health app use.[136] Stress was the most common mental health concern (44% of participants experienced stress); the more someone experiences stress, the more likely they are to use a mental health app. Perceived need for help was associated with mental health app use, and the use of the mental health app predicated on its being free, private, and would include others with similar situations. Past use of services, like seeing a counselor, was strongly associated with mental health app use.

In addition, privacy concerns were related to nonuse of a mental health app.[137] Social influence (other peoples' opinions of mental health app use) was associated with higher mental health app use. Finally, perceived need strongly mediated the effect of perceived stress on mental health app usage.

There were several implications to Borghouts et al.'s work.[138] First, to promote mental health app usage, the app should be free, private, and encouraged. Second, help-seeking should be normalized. Third, counselors and other campus personnel should promote and encourage app use. And finally, student endorsement of app use and effectiveness could be helpful to increase usage among other students.

## Coping Strategies

Tori I. Rehr and David J. Nguyen argued that "[c]ommunity college student affairs professionals are . . . in need of evidence-based tools to build collaborative mental health programming most applicable to their students."[139] Accordingly, they aimed to determine "which coping styles community college students use and the correlation of those behaviors with common mental health concerns."[140] These authors focused on community college students who had accessed a community college counseling center. The focus was on approach and avoidance coping.

According to Rehr and Nguyen, "community college students are particularly likely to use self-blame and problem-solving coping styles at the time of their first counseling session. Additionally, avoidance coping mechanism (i.e., self-blame, substance use, and disengagement) are correlated with anxiety and depression symptomatology."[141]

Within this study, there was a high rate of healthy coping behaviors among community college students.[142] But participants of this study *were going to counseling*. And some coping strategies may work better than others within a community college context. Furthermore, Rehr and Nguyen encouraged practitioners to conceptualize certain coping strategies, such as substance use, self-blame, and disengagement, "as largely maladaptive in the academic context."[143]

The authors also noted that "[g]iven the potentially severe impacts on mental health, self-blame coping should be a particular area of focus for mental health professionals and other [community college] campus personnel."[144] Community college personnel ought to provide students information about adaptive coping mechanisms and move students away from using self-blame to cope. This has been shown to work well in other contexts.[145] Lastly, it should also be noted that students who use adaptive coping mechanisms may *also* be using maladaptive ones.

## Evaluations of Campus Interventions or Actions

Some of the literature on community college student mental health is focused on the evaluation of campus interventions or actions. Two such examples include web-based interactions and peer-to-peer support programming.

## Web-based Interventions

Web-based interventions (WBIs) may assist with the following problem: mental health issues are more prevalent among community college students than students at four-year institutions, yet community college students have access to fewer on-campus mental health resources than their counterparts at four-year institutions. Liza N. Meredith and Patricia A. Frazier examined the effectiveness of a web-based stress management program across a sample of community college students. Specifically, the stress management program focused on increasing present control, which the authors explained "focuses on current thoughts, feelings, and behaviors" by asking the question, for example, "Do I have control over how I deal with this event in the present?"[146] Present control was a focus area for their study because it has been shown to consistently predict positive mental health.

In their study, data on student participants were collected preintervention, postintervention, and three weeks after the intervention. Three relevant findings emerged. First, present control significantly increased from pre- to postintervention and from preintervention to the three-week follow up. Second, perceived stress significantly decreased from pre- to postintervention and from preintervention to the three-week follow up. And third, stress significantly decreased from pre- to postintervention and from preintervention to the three-week follow-up.[147]

The authors noted that the present control-focused stress management program was intended for use at four-year institutions, and it should be modified for the community college environment.[148] In sum, they argued "online interventions may be an affordable way to disseminate mental health information to students."[149] These WBIs should be recommended, not required, to students by community college personnel. These interventions may be especially helpful for students who are experiencing stress or are overwhelmed.

### Peer-to-Peer Support

While peer-to-peer mental health support initiatives have utility on four-year institution campuses, its promise is yet to be realized within the community college. In fact, there is almost no research on this topic. Before implementation, however, how peers respond to someone in distress must be known.

Enter Michael T. Kalkbrenner's work.[150] The Mental Distress Response Scale (MDRS) was administered to community college students to address this knowledge gap. It delineates two primary responses to a peer in mental health distress: diminish/avoid and approach/encourage. The purpose of the study was to test the MDRS across a number of subpopulations of community college students, including, gender, ethnicity, generational status, and help-seeking history."[151]

This study provided support for the reliability and validity of this scale with community college students.[152] Furthermore, it "found support for the utility of the MDRS for use with a number of demographic subpopulations of community college students."[153] This is important given the heterogeneity of community college students across the sector and across most community college campuses. Other interesting findings emerged. For example, non-white students in the study were less likely to respond to a peer in mental health distress. Specific interventions based on student subpopulation may be necessary to support all students.

Because the MDRS is short (only 10 items), it could easily be administered to community college students during new student orientation. The data could be used to build and evaluate a peer-to-peer mental health support initiative. Campus agents should use the data to promote approach/encourage behaviors. Based on the results of this study, the author argued that it may be good to recruit "counseling referral agents among students who have participated in personal counseling."[154]

Another example of a peer-to-peer support model happened during the 2020–2021 academic year at four community colleges in the San Francisco Bay Area.[155] These colleges piloted a mental health navigators program. Ten students (from social work, nursing, and social sciences) served as navigators. The fall semester was focused on learning about mental health topics, and the spring semester was focused on experiential learning. Students were given a small caseload of other students to help connect them to services in the local area. While the California Community Colleges (CCC) offer mental health services, the need usually surpasses what is available.

The CCC provides mental health services on a limited basis; students may have six to eight sessions per semester. Need outweighs available personnel, however. Students are referred to outside services but may have trouble navigating access and health insurance considerations. This led to the creation of this program, which is meant to help students continue receiving services (and to remain in college).

The authors outlined promising results, as determined by the retention of the 19 students who were part of the navigators' caseload.[156] It should be emphasized that the authors noted this project was not meant to be a research study, per se. In some ways, the pandemic paved the way for virtual learning and telehealth services. Students in the program showed high levels of satisfaction.

Sang Leng Trieu and Richard Chen's work provides an invaluable blueprint on how to develop such a program.[157] Sets of challenges and potential solutions to those challenges were provided. First, there was attrition among navigators; low enrollment, interest, and involvement were issues. Therefore, infrastructure should be built. Second, there were a low number of referrals from campus-based mental health therapists. This was from low interest among students and issues with the hand-off. As such, work should be done on relationships between the two groups, or dyads. Third, there was a need for more training and practice among navigators. There are two ways to address this: increase training and practice opportunities and add pandemic-based contextual information.

## SUMMARY

Most of the literature presented within this chapter was published during the past decade. Yet it will soon move into the canonical background. Ongoing interest and inquiry in this area is fully anticipated and necessary. The mental health impacts of the global COVID-19 pandemic are now beginning to emerge within the peer-reviewed literature, in which a time-lag is always embedded.[158] As this literature base matures, practitioners will have more knowledge from which to build support for students. Yet, there is so much that can be done now and in the future in consideration of what is already known. More on that to come.

Even though this chapter was built from a scoping review of the literature on community college student mental health, there remains a lot of work to do in this area. The research on college student mental health is nearly exclusively focused on the four-year sector. What is known about the community college sector shows its significance as a contemporary and enduring issue community college leaders must acknowledge and address—at least to some degree.

When students are struggling with mental health issues, achieving academic goals becomes more difficult. Supporting student mental health is another way institutions can remove barriers or assist students around or through barriers to their success. This is good for students, and, in turn, it is good for institutions. In fact, there is some evidence to suggest supporting students' mental health is good for institutional business.

The investment is worth it, especially considering students with symptoms of a mental health problem are twice as likely to leave college without graduating.[159] Supporting community college students is not just about individual success. This is an institutional, economic, and societal imperative. Individual community college student success transcends the individual.

When an individual student succeeds (i.e., earns a credential), institutional, economic, and societal benefits follow.[160] In fact, Ketchen Lipson et al. said "there is a strong economic case for federal, state, and local investments in the mental health of community college students through programs and services aimed at treatment and prevention and for social support services that could reduce financial stress."[161]

Within this chapter, recommendations given by the authors of the studies were profiled. These recommendations should be considered. The next six chapters are built from the study I conducted on this topic. The book then concludes with two chapters focused on recommendations based on that study and the literature presented in this chapter.

## NOTES

1. American Association of Community Colleges, "2022 Fast Facts," https://www.aacc.nche.edu/2022/02/28/42888/.

2. Paula E. McBride, "Addressing the Lack of Mental Health Services for At-Risk Students at a Two-Year Community College: A Contemporary Review," *Community College Journal of Research and Practice* 43, no. 2 (2019), 146–148, https://doi.org/10.1080/10668926.2017.1409670.

3. McBride, "Addressing the Lack of Mental Health Services."

4. Danielle Melidona, Morgan Taylor, and Ty C. McNamee, *Fall 2021 Term Pulse Points Survey of College and University Presidents* (Washington, DC: American Council on Education. October 25, 2021), https://www.acenet.edu/Research-Insights/Pages/Senior-Leaders/Presidents-Survey-Fall-2021.aspx.

5. Kasey Edwardson, "Quantitative Approaches to Community College Student Health: A Systematic Review of the Literature," *Community College Journal of Research and Practice* 45, no. 6 (2020): 451–462, https://doi.org/10.1080/10668926.2020.1722293.

6. Edwardson, "Quantitative Approaches."

7. Daniel Eisenberg et al., *Too Distressed to Learn? Mental Health among Community College Students* (Washington, DC: ACCT, 2016), https://www.acct.org/product/too-distressed-learn-mental-health-among-community-college-students-2016.

8. Eisenberg et al., *Too Distressed to Learn?*

9. Eisenberg et al., *Too Distressed to Learn?*, 2.

10. Sarah Ketchen Lipson et al., "Mental Health Conditions Among Community College Students: A National Study of Prevalence and Use of Treatment Services," *Psychiatric Services* 72, no. 10 (October 2021): 1126–1133, https://doi.org/10.1176/appi.ps.202000437.

11. Ketchen Lipson et al., "Mental Health Conditions," 1129.

12. Ketchen Lipson et al., "Mental Health Conditions," 1129.

13. Ketchen Lipson et al., "Mental Health Conditions," 1127.

14. Ketchen Lipson et al., "Mental Health Conditions," 1127.

15. Ketchen Lipson et al., "Mental Health Conditions."

16. Edwardson, "Quantitative Approaches," 2.

17. Sarah B. Oswalt et al., "Trends in College Students' Mental Health Diagnoses and Utilization of Services, 2009–2015," *Journal of American College Health* 68, no. 1 (2020): 41–51. https://doi.org/10.1080/07448481.2018.1515748.

18. Oswalt et al., "Trends in College Students' Mental Health," 44.

19. Oswalt et al., "Trends in College Students' Mental Health," 45.

20. Oswalt et al., "Trends in College Students' Mental Health," 48.

21. Jennifer M. Cadigan, Jennifer C. Duckworth, and Christine M. Lee, "Physical and Mental Health Issues Facing Community College Students," *Journal of American*

*College Health* 70, no. 3 (2020): 891–897, http://doi.org/10.1080/07448481.2020.1776716.

22. Cadigan et al., "Physical and Mental Health Issues," 891.

23. Cadigan et al., "Physical and Mental Health Issues."

24. Cadigan et al., "Physical and Mental Health Issues," 896.

25. Daniel Seth Katz and Karen Davison, "Community College Student Mental Health: A Comparative Analysis," *Community College Review* 42, no. 4 (October 2014): 307–26, https://doi.org/10.1177/0091552114535466.

26. Katz and Davison, "Community College Mental Health," 319.

27. Katz and Davison, "Community College Mental Health," 319.

28. Monica L. Heller and Jerrell C. Cassady, "Predicting Community College and University Student Success: A Test of the Triadic Reciprocal Model for Two Populations," *Journal of College Student Retention: Research, Theory, & Practice* 18, no. 4 (2015): 431–456. https://www.doi.org/10.1177/1521025115611130.

29. Heller and Cassady, "Predicting Community College."

30. Heller and Cassady, "Predicting Community College," 445.

31. Heller and Cassady, "Predicting Community College," 446.

32. Heller and Cassady, "Predicting Community College," 446; Urie Bronfenbrenner, "Toward an Experimental Ecology of Human Development," *American Psychologist*, 32, no. 7 (1977): 513–531, https://doi.org/10.1037/0003–066X.32.7.513.

33. Heller and Cassady, "Predicting Community College," 446.

34. Heller and Cassady, "Predicting Community College."

35. Daniel Eisenberg, Justin Hunt, and Nicole Speer, "Mental Health in American Colleges and Universities: Variation Across Student Subgroups and Across Campuses," *The Journal of Nervous and Mental Disease* 201, no. 1 (January 2013): 60–67, https://www.doi.org/10.1097/NMD.0b013e31827ab077.

36. Eisenberg, Hunt, and Speer, "Mental Health in American Colleges and Universities," 60.

37. Rachel J. Voth Schrag and Tonya E. Edmond, "Intimate Partner Violence, Trauma, and Mental Health Need Among Female Community College Students," *Journal of American College Health* 66, no. 7 (2018): 702–711, https://doi.org/10.1080/07448481.2018.1456443.

38. Voth Schrag and Edmond, "Intimate Partner Violence," 702.

39. Voth Schrag and Edmond, "Intimate Partner Violence," 707.

40. Voth Schrag and Edmond, "Intimate Partner Violence."

41. Voth Schrag and Edmond, "Intimate Partner Violence."

42. Voth Schrag and Edmond, "Intimate Partner Violence," 709.

43. Voth Schrag and Edmond, "Intimate Partner Violence," 708.

44. Voth Schrag and Edmond, "Intimate Partner Violence."

45. Voth Schrag and Edmond, "Intimate Partner Violence," 709.

46. Rebecca M. Howard et al., "Sexual Violence Victimization Among Community College Students," *Community College Journal of Research and Practice* 67, no. 7 (2019): 674–687, https://doi.org/10.1080/07448481.2018.1500474.

47. Howard et al., "Sexual Violence Victimization."

48. Howard et al., "Sexual Violence Victimization."

49. Howard et al., "Sexual Violence Victimization."

50. Howard et al., "Sexual Violence Victimization."

51. Emily A. Pierceall and Maybelle C. Keim, "Stress and Coping Strategies Among Community College Students," *Community College Journal of Research and Practice* 31, no. 9 (2007): 703–712, https://doi.org/10.1080/10668920600866579.

52. Pierceall and Keim, "Stress and Coping Strategies."

53. Pierceall and Keim, "Stress and Coping Strategies."

54. Paris Scott Strom et al., "Gender Differences in Stress of Community College Students," *Community College Journal of Research and Practice* 46, no. 7 (2022): 472–487, https://www.doi.org/10.1080/10668926.2021.1873872.

55. Strom et al., "Gender Differences in Stress."

56. Strom et al., "Gender Differences in Stress."

57. Strom et al., "Gender Differences in Stress."

58. Laura Martin and Lynn Bohecker, "Community College Student Well-Being and Implications For Care," *Community College Journal of Research and Practice* 46, no. 8 (2021): 560–572, https://doi.org/10.1080/10668926.2021.1883487.

59. Martin and Bohecker, "Community College Student Well-Being."

60. John C. Fortney et al., "Mental Health Treatment Seeking Among Veteran and Civilian Community College Students," *Psychiatric Services* 68, no. 8 (2017): 851–855, https://doi.org/10.1176/appi.ps.201600240.

61. Fortney et al., "Mental Health Treatment Seeking," 851.

62. Fortney et al., "Mental Health Treatment Seeking."

63. Fortney et al., "Mental Health Treatment Seeking," 854.

64. Fortney et al., "Mental Health Treatment Seeking," 854.

65. Fortney et al., "Mental Health Treatment Seeking," 854.

66. Meekyung Han and Helen Pong, "Mental Health Help-Seeking Behaviors Among Asian American Community College Students: The Effects of Stigma, Cultural Barriers, and Acculturation," *Journal of College Student Development* 56, no. 1 (January 2015): 1–14, https://doi.org/10.1353/csd.2015.0001.

67. Han and Pong, "Mental Health Help-Seeking Behaviors."

68. Jeanne L. Edman, Susan B. Watson, and David J. Patron, "Trauma and Psychological Distress Among Ethnically Diverse Community College Students," *Community College Journal of Research and Practice* 40, no. 4 (2016): 336, http://dx.doi.org/10.1080/10668926.2015.1065211.

69. Edman et al., "Trauma and Psychological Distress."

70. Edman et al., "Trauma and Psychological Distress."

71. Emalinda McSpadden, "I'm Not Crazy or Anything: Exploring Culture, Mental Health Stigma, and Mental Health Service Use Among Urban Community College Students," *Community College Journal of Research and Practice* 46, no. 3 (2021): 202–214, https://doi.org/10.1080/10668926.2021.1922321.

72. McSpadden, "I'm Not Crazy or Anything."

73. McSpadden, "I'm Not Crazy or Anything," 212.

74. Jennifer M. Cadigan and Christine M. Lee, "Identifying Barriers to Mental Health Service Utilization Among Heavy Drinking Community College Students,"

*Community College Journal of Research and Practice* 43, no. 8 (2019): 585–594, https://doi.org/10.1080/10668926.2018.1520659.

75. Cadigan and Lee, "Identifying Barriers," 587.

76. Cadigan and Lee, "Identifying Barriers."

77. Cadigan and Lee, "Identifying Barriers."

78. Cadigan and Lee, "Identifying Barriers," 591.

79. Cadigan and Lee, "Identifying Barriers," 592.

80. Stacy Waters-Bailey, Matthew S. McGraw, and Jason Barr, "Serving the Whole Student: Addressing Nonacademic Barriers Facing Rural Community College Students," *New Directions for Community Colleges* 2019, no. 187 (Fall 2019): 83–93, https://www.doi.org/10.1002/cc.20372.

81. Waters-Bailey et al., "Serving the Whole Student," 83.

82. Waters-Bailey et al., "Serving the Whole Student."

83. Waters-Bailey et al., "Serving the Whole Student," 91.

84. Lesley Rennis et al., "Google It!: Urban Community College Students' Use of the Internet to Obtain Self-Care and Personal Health Information," *College Student Journal* 46, no. 3 (Fall 2015): 414–426, https://www.ingentaconnect.com/content/prin/csj/2015/00000049/00000003/art00010.

85. Rennis et al., "Google It!," 422.

86. Rennis et al., "Google It!," 425.

87. American Association of Community Colleges (AACC), "Fast Facts 2022," Research Trends, revised May 11, 2022, https://www.aacc.nche.edu/research-trends/fast-facts/.

88. Divya P. Shenoy, Christine Lee, and Sang Leng Trieu, "The Mental Health Status of Single-Parent Community College Students in California," *Journal of American College Health* 64, no. 2 (2016): 152–156, https://dx.doi.org/10.1080/07448481.2015.1057147.

89. Shenoy et al., "The Mental Health Status," 155.

90. Shenoy et al., "The Mental Health Status," 156.

91. Shenoy et al., "The Mental Health Status," 155.

92. National Junior College Athletic Association, "Compete NJCAA," https://www.njcaa.org/compete/index.

93. Joshua C. Watson, "The Effect of Athletic Identity and Locus of Control on the Stress Perceptions of Community College Student-Athletes," *Community College Journal of Research and Practice* 40, no. 9 (2016): 729–738, https://doi.org/10.1080/10668926.2015.1072595.

94. Watson, "The Effect of Athletic Identity."

95. Watson, "The Effect of Athletic Identity."

96. Watson, "The Effect of Athletic Identity," 735.

97. Watson, "The Effect of Athletic Identity."

98. Laura Brogden and Dennis E. Gregory, "Resilience in Community College Students with Adverse Childhood Experiences," *Community College Journal of Research and Practice* 43, no. 2 (2019): 94–108, https://doi.org/10.1080/10668926.2017.1418685.

99. Brodgen and Gregory, "Resilience in Community College Students," 100.

100. Brodgen and Gregory, "Resilience in Community College Students."

101. Brodgen and Gregory, "Resilience in Community College Students."

102. Joan B. Hirt, *Where You Work Matters: Student Affairs Administration at Different Types of Institutions* (Lanham, MD: University Press of America, 2006).

103. Kenneth M. Coll and Reese M. House, "Empirical Implications for the Training and Development of Community College Counselors," *Community College Review* 19, no. 2 (Fall 1991): 43–52, https://doi.org/10.1177/009155219101900207.

104. Coll and House, "Empirical Implications."

105. Coll and House, "Empirical Implications."

106. Coll and House, "Empirical Implications."

107. Beth A. Durodoye, Henry L. Harris, and Vernie L. Bolden, "Personal Counseling as a Function of the Community College Counseling Experience," *Community College Review* 24, no. 6 (2000): 455–468, https://doi.org/10.1080/10668920050137237.

108. For more information on extant counseling centers on community college campuses, see this report: American College Counseling Association (ACCA) Community College Task Force, *Survey of Community/2 Year College Counseling Services*, 2011, https://www.sbctc.edu/resources/documents/about/task-forces-work-groups/ctc-counselors/acca-national-survey-of-community-college-counseling-services.pdf.

109. Michelle Dykes-Anderson, "The Case for Comprehensive Counseling Centers at Community Colleges," *Community College Journal of Research and Practice* 37, no. 10 (2013): 742–749, https://www.doi.org/10.1080/10668921003723235.

110. Dykes-Anderson, "The Case for Comprehensive Counseling Centers."

111. Dykes-Anderson, "The Case for Comprehensive Counseling Centers," 745.

112. Dykes-Anderson, "The Case for Comprehensive Counseling Centers."

113. Danna Ethan and Erica J. Seidel, "On the Front Lines of Student Crisis: Urban Community College Professors' Experiences and Perceived Role in Handling Students in Distress," *College Student Affairs Journal* 31 no. 1 (Spring 2013): 15–26.

114. Ethan and Seidel, "On the Front Lines," 16.

115. Ethan and Seidel, "On the Front Lines," 19.

116. Ethan and Seidel, "On the Front Lines," 21.

117. Ethan and Seidel, "On the Front Lines," 22.

118. Ethan and Seidel, "On the Front Lines," 22.

119. Ethan and Seidel, "On the Front Lines."

120. Mike Kalkbrenner and Thomas J. Hernández, "Community Colleges Students' Awareness of Risk Factors for Mental Health Problems and Referrals to Facilitative and Debilitative Resources," *Community College Journal of Research and Practice* 41, no. 1 (2017): 56–64, https://doi.org/10.1080/10668926.2016.1179603.

121. Kalkbrenner and Hernández, "Community Colleges Students' Awareness," 59.

122. Kalkbrenner and Hernández, "Community Colleges Students' Awareness," 60.

123. Michael T. Kalkbrenner, "Recognizing and Supporting Students with Mental Health Disorders: The REDFLAGS Model," *Journal of Education and Training* 3, no. 1 (February 2016), http://dx.doi.org/10.5296/jet.v3i1.8141.

124. Michael T. Kalkbrenner et al., "Utility of the REDFLAGS Model for Supporting Community College Students' Mental Health: Implications for Counselors," *Journal of Counseling and Development* 97, no. 4 (October 2019): 418, https://doi.org/10.1002/jcad.12290.

125. Kalkbrenner et al., "Utility of the REDFLAGS Model."

126. Kalkbrenner et al., "Utility of the REDFLAGS Model," 423.

127. Kalkbrenner et al., "Utility of the REDFLAGS Model."

128. Sarah Ketchen Lipson et al., "Mental Health Conditions Among Community College Students: A National Study of Prevalence and Use of Treatment Services," *Psychiatric Services* 72, no. 10 (October 2021): 1129, https://doi.org/10.1176/appi.ps.202000437.

129. Michael S. Dunbar et al., "Unmet Mental Health Treatment Need and Attitudes Toward Online Mental Health Services Among Community College Students," *Psychiatric Services* 69, no. 5 (May 1, 2018): 597, https://doi.org/10.1176/appi.ps.201700402.

130. Dunbar et al., "Unmet Mental Health Treatment Need," 598.

131. Judith Borghouts et al., "Understanding Mental Health App Use Among Community College Students: Web-Based Survey Study," *Journal of Medical Internet Research* 23, no. 9 (2021): e27745, https://www.doi.org/10.2196/27745.

132. Borghouts et al., "Understanding Mental Health App Use."

133. Borghouts et al., "Understanding Mental Health App Use," para 4.

134. Borghouts et al., "Understanding Mental Health App Use."

135. Borghouts et al., "Understanding Mental Health App Use."

136. Borghouts et al., "Understanding Mental Health App Use."

137. Borghouts et al., "Understanding Mental Health App Use."

138. Borghouts et al., "Understanding Mental Health App Use."

139. Tori I. Rehr and David J. Nguyen, "Approach/Avoidance Coping Among Community College Students and Applications for Student Affairs Professionals," *Journal of Student Affairs Research and Practice* 59, no. 3 (2021): 238, https://doi.org/10.1080/19496591.2021.1914641.

140. Rehr and Nguyen, "Approach/Avoidance Coping," 238.

141. Rehr and Nguyen, "Approach/Avoidance Coping," 238.

142. Rehr and Nguyen, "Approach/Avoidance Coping."

143. Rehr and Nguyen, "Approach/Avoidance Coping," 247.

144. Rehr and Nguyen, "Approach/Avoidance Coping," 247.

145. See, for example, Janaina L. Fogaca, "Combining Mental Health and Performance Interventions: Coping and Social Support for Student-Athletes," *Journal of Applied Sport Psychology* 33, no. 1 (2019): 4–19, https://doi.org/10.1080/10413200.2019.1648326.

146. Meredith and Frazier, "Randomized Trial," 43.

147. Meredith and Frazier, "Randomized Trial."

148. Meredith and Frazier, "Randomized Trial."

149. Meredith and Frazier, "Randomized Trial," 53.

150. Michael T. Kalkbrenner, "Peer-to-Peer Mental Health Support on Community College Campuses: Examining the Factorial Invariance of the Mental Distress

Response Scale," *Community College Journal of Research and Practice* 44, no. 10–12 (2020): 757–770, https://doi.org/10.1080/10668926.2019.1645056.

151. Kalkbrenner, "Peer-to-Peer Mental Health Support," 760.

152. Kalkbrenner, "Peer-to-Peer Mental Health Support."

153. Kalkbrenner, "Peer-To-Peer Mental Health Support," 766.

154. Kalkbrenner, "Peer-to-Peer Mental Health Support," 768.

155. Sang Leng Trieu and Richard Chen, "Community College Mental Health Navigators: A Pilot Program to Improve Access to Care," *Health Promotion Practice* (2022):1–4, https://doi.org/10.1177/15248399221090917.

156. Leng Trieu and Chen, "Community College Mental Health Navigators."

157. Leng Trieu and Chen, "Community College Mental Health Navigators."

158. See, for example, JoAnne Bullard, "Preparing for a Return to Play: Understanding the Impact of COVID-19 on the Well-Being of Community College Student-Athletes," *Community College Journal of Research and Practice* 46, no. 3 (2022): 215–222, https://doi.org/10.1080/10668926.2021.1982796; Jacquelyn Chin et al., "'I Help My Parents by Using Some of My FAFSA Money': A Qualitative Exploration of Pandemic-Related Stress Among Community College Students," *Community College Journal of Research and Practice* (2022), https://doi.org/10.1080/10668926.2022.2064376.

159. Daniel Eisenberg, Ezra Golberstein, and Justin B. Hunt, "Mental Health and Academic Success in College," *The B.E. Journal of Economic Analysis & Policy* 9, no. 1 (2009): Article 40, http://www.bepress.com/bejeap/vol9/iss1/art40.

160. Clive Belfield and Davis Jenkins, *Community College Economics for Policymakers: One Big Fact and One Big Myth* (Working Paper No. 67, New York, NY: Community College Research Center (CCRC), 2014), https://ccrc.tc.columbia.edu/media/k2/attachments/community-college-economics-for-policymakers.pdf.

161. Ketchen Lipson et al., "Mental Health Conditions," 1131.

# PART II

# The Faculty

The two chapters within this section are meant to introduce the faculty who participated in this study. Chapter 4 first includes an overview of the study and then is focused on the participants' faculty career pathways, dispositions, and pedagogies. Getting a sense of how participants arrived at their faculty positions, their orientations to education, and their approaches to and strategies for teaching is important to understanding their perceptions of and experiences with their students' mental health.

Faculty commentary on their students' assets and obstacles are then presented in chapter 5. Resilience was asserted as a major asset among students, while finances were overwhelmingly noted as students' biggest obstacle. Resiliency is forged through enduring difficulty, and many community college students have endured significant life challenges. Living in poverty and experiencing financial stress are related to mental health issues. As such, this section sets the stage for what follows.

Within this section and the one that follows, some long excerpts from the interviews are included verbatim so the richness of the data comes through. Engaging with these professionals was a sincere privilege. Their voices are highlighted herein and extended meaning of their insights are made through interpretation. Moreover, the extant literature is also used throughout the next six chapters to help situate participants' voices within what is already known.

## Chapter 4

# Career Pathways, Dispositions, and Pedagogies

"I love it [teaching], and I love my job, and I love my classes. I love what I teach. I love my students."

–Sandie

As the first section of this book made clear, the mental health of community college students is an increasingly critical issue. Furthermore, to deeply understand the issue, the perspectives of community college faculty are essential. That is where this book steps in. This chapter houses details about the study undergirding this book and the backgrounds, career pathways, dispositions, and pedagogies of the community college faculty participants of the study. Note that a fuller treatment of the study's research design is presented in Appendix A.

As student mental health issues began to emerge as a problem anecdotally and in the literature (see chapter 3), in early 2017, 22 community college faculty members were interviewed about their perceptions of and experiences with their students' mental health. All participants were employed at the same community college in the mid-Atlantic region of the United States with several campuses.

Of the 22 faculty, 19 were women and only three were men. This overrepresentation of women was also the case with similar studies.[1] There were no transgender, gender nonbinary, or gender nonconforming participants. All faculty identified as white. The youngest participant was 29, the oldest was 69—a 40-year span. The average age was 51.5; the median age was 56.5. The person with the shortest tenure at the institution was less than a year, while the person with the longest had been employed there for 28 years. Fifteen faculty members were employed full-time, while seven were part-time, or adjunct.

All participants had experience teaching in-person, and some had experience teaching online. Many different subject areas were represented such as developmental reading and writing, legal studies, art history, sonography, nursing, and early childhood education.

It should be noted that the participants in the study were not necessarily representative of the faculty population at the institution. For example, while 68 percent of the faculty sample were full-time, only 15 percent of the institution's full faculty are full-time. And the characteristics of the faculty interviewed certainly have some bearing on the insights they provided. That all participants are white must be accounted for, especially considering just 65 percent of the student body are white.

Interpretations of how faculty characteristics informed their work and what was shared within the interviews is provided through the chapters that follow, yet readers should also keep this context in mind when considering those interpretations. See chapter 1 and Appendix A for more details. For the purposes of maintaining the institution's identity and participants' identities confidential, a full articulation of the study's context is withheld. A complete picture of the faculty members who participated in the study is below in table 4.1.

Within this section and the next, the hope is for readers to feel as though they *know* the faculty participants whose generosity with their time and insight gave way to this text. As such, robust description and ample inclusion of verbatim excerpts from the interviews are included. Much of what follows will, hopefully, bring to life the participants' vibrantly articulated perceptions and experiences related to community college student mental health. The interviews started with questions meant to get to know and build rapport with participants. The sections that follow include career pathways, dispositions, and pedagogies—all of which informed their perceptions and experiences.

Career pathways refers to the routes taken by faculty to arrive in their teaching positions at the community college. Dispositions refer to faculty ways of being as educators. To borrow a term from philosophy, disposition could also be seen as participants' pedagogical *ontologies*. It is *who they are* as faculty in relation to their teaching. Disposition was also connected to purpose. In other words, their dispositions were informed, in part, by their purpose. Their purpose drove *why* they did what they did as educators.

Finally, pedagogy refers to teaching approaches, strategies, and behaviors. It was difficult to tease out the differences between dispositions and pedagogies, as they are intertwined and mutually informed. Knowing where participants are coming from in addition to *who they are*, *what they do*, and *why they do it* provides scaffolding for understanding the insights they brought to this study.

**Table 4.1. Faculty Participants' Information**

| Participant Pseudonym | Subject(s) Taught | Employment Status | Perception of % of Students with Mental Health Issues | Years Employed at Institution (total) | Highest Degree (self-report) | Gender | Race | Age |
|---|---|---|---|---|---|---|---|---|
| Pam | Nursing | Full-time | 25% | 8 | Doctorate | Woman | White | 31 |
| Carolyn | Developmental English | Full-time | 30% | 19 | Doctoral | Woman | White | 67 |
| Tess | Business | Adjunct | 60-70% | <1 | MBA | Woman | White | 29 |
| Sandie | Developmental English, Business Writing, Technical Communication | Adjunct | ("at least") 50% | 3.5 | Master's | Woman | White | 46 |
| Eve | Art History | Full-time | "it's huge" | 17 | Doctorate | Woman | White | 48 |
| Suzie | Developmental English (writing); English | Full-time | "pretty prevalent" | 6 | Ph.D. | Woman | White | 63 |
| Ken | Respiratory Therapy | Full-time | No direct answer | 15 | Master's | Man | White | 49 |
| Rebecca | Developmental English (reading); First-Year Seminar | Part-time | "very prevalent" | 10 | Master's | Woman | White | 58 |
| Helen | Psychology | Full-time | "Oh, it's rampant." | 17 | Master's | Woman | White | 56 |
| Camille | Early Childhood and Elementary Education | Full-time | "I think that they [mental health concerns] are there." | Approx. 25 | Master's | Woman | White | 59 |

| Name | Subject | Status | Prevalence | Gender | Race | Age | Experience/Degree |
|---|---|---|---|---|---|---|---|
| Martin | Developmental English (reading and composition) | Full-time | No direct answer; more prevalent than he thought | Man | White | 46 | 14 Master's |
| Joy | Human Services; Social Work | Part-time | "It's fairly prevalent." | Woman | White | 59 | 28 Master's |
| Sophie | Biology; Foundations (First-Year Seminar) | Part-time | "I think there's a lot, a lot of issues going on." | Woman | White | 38 | 6 Master's |
| Jody | Nursing | Part-time | 10% | Woman | White | 62 | 16 Master's |
| Harriet | English | Full-time | more than before; with more severity | Woman | White | 68 | 15 Master's |
| Marie | Biology | Full-time | No direct answer | Woman | White | 62 | 17 Master's |
| Rose | Psychology | Full-time | "quite prevalent" | Woman | White | 69 | 18 Ph.D. |
| Phoebe | Legal Studies | Full-time | "pretty prevalent" | Woman | White | 52 | 15 JD |
| Christina | Sonography | Full-time | "Huge." | Woman | White | 57 | 13 Bachelor's |
| Stephanie | Foundational Studies | Full-time | "very prevalent" "at least one-third of my students" | Woman | White | 44 | 16 Master's |

| Geraldine | Developmental English (reading) | Full-time | "every class" | 16 Master's | Woman | White | 52 |
| Justin | Human Services (Sociology) | Adjunct | "I think it's a huge issue." | 17 Master's | Man | White | 57 |

## CAREER PATHWAYS

Many community college faculty *end up in*, *land in*, or *fall into* their teaching positions rather than actively seek them out.[2] And for those who do want to teach at the college level, many aspire to teach at the four-year level. Sometimes employment is gained through applying for positions, while others may be shoulder-tapped or asked to apply for certain positions. Some may transition from the K-12 space.

Still others may have a connection to the institution, link to a specific program, or experience as an adjunct and move into a full-time faculty position. Some may have been a community college student. For others, teaching at the community college for the first time may be their first meaningful experience within the community college environment. Some who begin in part-time positions find they really enjoy the work and the sector and therefore want to shift into full-time teaching.

Others prefer to teach on a part-time basis. Many adjunct faculty are happily employed within the field and may teach a class or two to give back to the profession. Working at the community college in a teaching-adjacent capacity is also a pathway to a faculty role. Those with experience working within learning or tutoring centers, for example, may be strong candidates for teaching developmental education courses. The backgrounds and career pathways of participants informed their faculty work. Below are examples of participants' career pathways into community college teaching. These examples demonstrate the diversity of career backgrounds.

The oldest participant in the study at 69, Rose, did secretarial training in high school. She started college but left to help support her family, as her father died when she was 11 years old. She intended to earn a bachelor's degree, and she earned an associate's degree. She later got into pharmaceutical sales and moved around the country quite a bit. And moreover, she became a mother. After deciding to go back to school, she stayed for 11 years and earned a bachelor's degree, two master's degrees, and a Ph.D. She moved from general studies to sociology to psychology. Rose started teaching at the community college while pursuing her Ph.D.

Marie never anticipated teaching—even though both her parents were teachers. She started a Ph.D. after marrying and having children. But she then realized the lab setting was not working out well. So, she got a master's degree and started teaching at a community college in a neighboring state. She was later tapped for a position after moving to the area where she has been teaching biology for 17 years.

Phoebe was in a similar situation as Marie; she said, "I've never thought I would be teaching. It's really not what I aimed for." She graduated from law school with the intention of being a lawyer. She practiced as a lawyer and then got married, relocated, and had a child.

The transition to the new area was difficult, especially since she was only one of two female lawyers at her firm, and the first female lawyer to have children. She explained that her firm "really didn't know what to do with me" after she had her first child. She attempted to limit her hours at that time, but her firm still expected her to do as much work. She summarized, "So, it didn't work out too well." She then moved into contract work, including doing work in construction law. She then had a second child and stopped working.

But after 18 months, she started thinking about returning to work. Her husband had been teaching at the community college and was serving as a dean. He told her about the college needing faculty to teach courses geared for individuals who worked in construction and who wanted to become managers. The college had partnered with a local construction company to deliver these courses, and a faculty member with a law background was preferred. Phoebe recounted that her husband told her: "We're looking for a lawyer to teach it. I want you to teach it."

Phoebe was initially hesitant but eventually agreed. She was glad she did. She shared she "ended up really liking it [teaching]." That was the start of what turned into a fulfilling teaching career. After seven years of teaching part-time, the college decided to hire a full-time faculty member to oversee the paralegal program in 2007. After a nationwide search, Phoebe got the job.

Jody worked in healthcare as a nurse interested in disease prevention while also teaching at a private four-year institution where she built a strong reputation as a teacher. But the program closed. So, she then moved into the community college setting. Nursing faculty are in high demand, and she enjoyed the community college space, noting "the [student] work ethic is much more here" in comparison to her teaching experiences at a local, private, and selective four-year institution.

Christina worked as an X-ray technician—also doing ultrasound—until two shoulder injuries kept her from continuing. Therefore, she applied for a teaching position at the community college. She started out working with students, overseeing them at clinical sites. Then she moved into teaching upon earning her bachelor's degree. She said she "fell into teaching" and now directs clinical education, which suits her well considering her background.

A developmental English faculty member, Martin explained that he came to higher education "late." He also came to college teaching "late," working in hotel management earlier in his career. Martin was a student at the college and got his first position at the institution as a part-time tutor. He then moved into directing the Learning Center. This experience gives him good insights on student resources. He applied for and got a teaching position after finishing his master's degree. He reflected: "I never saw myself here [teaching at the community college]. But I think it's where I always should have been."

Like Martin, Stephanie started as a counselor for the college while adjuncting within foundational studies (i.e., first-year seminar courses). Prior to that, she worked in vocational rehabilitation after earning a master's degree in counseling. She then moved into a full-time teaching position within foundational studies.

Helen had full-time clinical work experience in the field and then became an adjunct, teaching psychology courses. Working as an adjunct led to a full-time position. She noted "[I] found that I really, really love teaching." She was ready to transition away from the clinical space and use what she learned there to inform her faculty work.

Similarly, Camille had lots of experience working in early childhood education prior to teaching it. She was asked to teach at the college while working on a master's degree. After adjuncting for a long time, she then moved into a full-time position once it was available. She explained being "very lucky" to have the opportunity to make this change.

Ken was a community college student at the institution after becoming a respiratory therapy equipment technician in high school. He has a personal story of triumph involving struggle, addiction, and recovery. He first worked as an adjunct while also working as a respiratory therapist after graduation. He also was pursuing his bachelor's degree at that time.

When the program's Director of Clinical Education role opened at the college, Ken had just finished his bachelor's degree, which made him eligible for the position and he got the job. In that role, he shared he "did a lot with the program." Later, when the program director retired, he then got that job. In many ways, his community college degree and experience gave him the foundation to "work [his] way up" and build a fulfilling career.

Ken, at the time of the interview, had two master's degrees and was working on a doctorate. His career pathway influences him as a teacher: "I guess because of my own experiences I very much believe in second chances, and I believe that people can overcome and I understand the trials and the struggles that are involved in that."

As seen within these career pathways, some faculty have entire careers before realizing their desire to teach. Some had others encourage them to pursue teaching opportunities. And over time, some realize the classroom is exactly where they want to be. Common to all participants was excitement about the work they do as faculty within the community college context. In the next section, faculty dispositions are the focus.

## DISPOSITIONS

These participants were a passionate lot—passionate about their teaching and, for many, the social justice work it afforded them. This passion came from the sense of purpose they felt and maintained in their work with students. Many community college students come from marginalized backgrounds and harbor (multiple) marginalized identities.

This was not lost on their faculty. Suzie explained: "for the first time for me, in America, I was working with the unprivileged, the ones who, you know, had gotten the short end of the stick. So, it really kind of kicked in. I, I'm not saying I'm a saint here, I don't mean to, but it [teaching at a community college] kicked in my social justice, I guess." Suzie had a sense of purpose related to social justice prior to teaching at the community college but recognizing her own privilege and reflecting on her context helped her sustain purpose and motivation within the faculty position.

Faculty widely expressed that the diversity among their students is the best part of their jobs. They reveled in it and rose to the opportunities and challenges it presented. The students with whom they worked were diverse in every way possible. And the faculty welcomed and relished that diversity. In fact, Rebecca shared "I love the diversity of students. I never imagined how fabulous that part would be." She spoke excitedly about how a diverse group of students could grow into a rich community. Joy added: "I like the students. I really like the diversity of the students and of all the things they bring to the table."

Camille also spoke at length about enjoying the diversity of her students and being able to support those students.

> By diversity I mean, everybody comes from a completely different environment, and they have different responsibilities. . . . The 1:10 class today, which is elementary ed[ucation], tend to be mostly 18–25-year-olds. And I enjoy them, but I love to . . . have 50-year-olds in the class. Uh, people that are from different ethnic backgrounds, people that are single with three kids. Somebody said, 'I have three children, I'm taking five courses, and working full time.' And I just looked at her. Her grades are fabulous! . . . I think the thing that I love the most is being—is that they come to me, and I can listen and support them.

She mentioned knowing nothing about counseling, but she certainly knew a lot about listening. This is an important point that will be examined later in the book.

Rose noted enjoying student diversity and had an empathic understanding of older students' experiences, which she often shared with them. There was a sense of solidarity within her discussion of older students. She explained:

I love the variety of students. I particularly love nontraditional [older] students because I was one myself. And I love telling them, "You can do it. Don't be afraid that you can't, you know, perform as well as the young people. 'Cause you're probably gonna have an easier time, you're probably gonna do better." Because, and I tell them, instead of—I remember when I went to college the first time, I was just trying to memorize all these facts that, you know, didn't have any application, so it didn't really have any meaning to me. And when I went back to school it was like I had all these a-ha experiences, and I was like "A-ha! So that's why this happens that way. So, okay, now I understand this and that." And, you know, I did better grade-wise and—just loved it so much. And so I like to share that, you know, with my nontraditional students especially when they just come here and they're worried that they're not gonna do well. And, and the other thing I like to tell them is "Don't beat yourself up because you're late. You're doing it now, pat yourself on the back."

Some faculty referenced student diversity in comparison to other institution types, such as private four-year institutions. Stephanie was an example. She noted:

I do love the diversity of the students. . . . I remember my second year I think, I was saying, "This is great. I love the diversity. It's—every day, it's something new. It's something different. But some day, I can see myself just going to work for some private school where the students are all the same and it's easy and blah, blah, blah." That has not happened. I'm not, I'm apparently not really looking for that.

The use of the word "easy" in Stephanie's quote was in reference to her perception of what it would be like to teach within private higher education. She thought she would prefer working with private school students, who she envisioned as largely homogenous and college ready. She thought it would be easier to teach in that type of environment. Over time, however, she realized she preferred working with a diverse student population and within an institution where she did *not* see the work always easy.

Participants were also interested in continuous improvement. This was framed as an engaging challenge of the work. Phoebe constantly tried to figure out whether her teaching was working. She said, "It's hard to know, is it me or is it them?" She was referring to whether her teaching was ineffective or if a student did not study enough. In continuation, she said:

That's the hard thing. It's like no matter how I twist myself . . . I'm just not sure, is it me? Is it because students aren't as prepared as they were? Is it just this class? Am I off this year? Is it time for me to retire now? I just don't know [laughs]. So that's the hardest thing.

She is committed to constant betterment as an effective teacher. Geraldine expressed a similar sentiment:

Always watching [in the classroom], I'm always watching. I pay attention to who seems to be getting it, who's not getting it, like what—what is the demeanor? . . . Always trying to figure out what's going on. I think I've always been innately curious about people. Like, I've always been a people person, as an educator—boy, I just don't remember not doing it. Although I think I do it probably more deliberately now. But I think it just comes from this innate "What's going on there, what's making you tick?" And sometimes they [students] let you know, sometimes they don't.

Student success stories were a joyful component of the interviews. Seeing students learn, develop, and grow was a source of fulfillment and professional purpose. Christina explained:

I have a lot of student success stories. My students are so fun. They're so fun. . . . I've just had students over the years that you think, "Boy, they're just never going to get it," and all of a sudden, it's like, BOOM, it hit them like a brick wall, they got it, and they took off.

In a similar vein, Justin wanted to do the work necessary so students see education as valuable to their lives. He shared the following:

I get that student in a community college, who's been through addiction, who's been through rehabs, who's been through mental health services, who's been through whatever. Or they started having children when they were fourteen. And they're now 30, and they have five kids and, you know what I mean? It's like—they're graduating high school and, you look, they're 30 years old, they have kids and they're [grandparents], really, my god. I have a woman in my class who had a baby last night, her ninth child, you know? . . . I find the whole thing very fascinating, frankly. I like working with the students. These, a lot of times, these are the guys who, in [city], for example, who went to [name of high school] which, you don't know what that is, but that's the inner-city school for [city], and you're thinking, "Oh my god, what's the big deal, this is [city]" [laughs]. I know it's not, uh, it's not a metropolis or anything but, but they do have an inner-city, and they do have a bad, you know, bad schools, and they do—and a lot of those guys just didn't have a chance. And, between peer pressure and teen pregnancy and drugs and all the other activities that go on in those environments, they're sort of waking up just now. To, uh, the idea that oh, okay, education is valuable and, um, I might be able to do that. And, and I think that, right there, is the kind of thing that hooks me. 'Cause I want to hook them.

By "hook them," he is referring to cultivating buy-in within the community college student success arena. He wants to show students the power and promise of a higher education. Like Christina, this was something that drove and motivated Justin. Literally seeing a perspective, piece of information, or connection click into focus for a student was powerful—the "hook."

These faculty saw themselves as much more than content experts, arbiters of the curriculum, or responsible for filling their students' minds with information. Geraldine expressed this beautifully:

> I think the day, if there ever was a day where we as college professionals, professors, or professionals, could say "You know, my responsibility is totally curriculum. My responsibility is the content. The stuff going on in their lives has no bearing on me." Those days are gone. They need to be gone. . . . I've listened to students, I've heard things, and I've said "Oh, this is more than I can handle," or I mean not handle, but "It's more than I have an expertise in." But I think we bear the responsibility of informing, informing ourselves about some of the issues [affecting students]. I think that that is our responsibility as a faculty member.

She noted that faculty are on a continuum with regards to this point of view on teaching. She said those who teach developmental courses, like her, usually have a background or training in education, so there is a more holistic approach to the teaching and learning process among those faculty. It should be noted that while those who teach developmental courses at Geraldine's campus may have a background or training in education, this is not ubiquitous nationally.

Whether taking a holistic view of teaching, supporting students at the margins of society, improving teaching practice, or getting students "hooked" on learning, each faculty member expressed a passion for and purpose around teaching within the community college. Their dispositions—*who* they are as educators—informed *why* they taught, *how* they approached teaching, and *what* they did in (and out of) the classroom, which is the focus of the next section.

## PEDAGOGIES

Teaching is at the core of community college faculty work. This is a benefit of the work, not a deterrent, which participants were aware of and took seriously. Marie explained, "I think I might have been okay at research, but uh, I think that I'm an effective teacher, so I think that I like the fact that that's what the focus is, is teaching rather than, you know, bringing in funding and research dollars."

Furthermore, nearly all participants exuded student-centered, affirming, inclusive, empathic, caring, affect-conscious, and relational pedagogies. Throughout the interviews, these faculty presented as student advocates and excellent teachers. They routinely offered students affirmation and validation.[3]

Most had high expectations and provided students with the necessary scaffolding to meet those expectations through being willing to work with students outside of class, point them to resources, and adjust instructional approaches as needed. Also, most participants expressed an enjoyment of teaching, and many said they loved it. Ken demonstrated this well in stating: "I very much enjoy teaching. . . . And I love it." Most participants expressed positivity and even love regarding the joy they experienced through teaching. That enjoyment and love certainly came through in their praxis.

Suzie explained "[As an older person] I still love teaching, I always have. . . . I still get a huge kick out of it. Did not want to come back this semester [interview was early in the spring term], but then, you never do, really. You know? And then you get in with the students, and it works." Though teaching can be tiring, being with the students and experiencing the joy of teaching reminds her to keep going—and keep coming back.

Similarly, Camille added: "I love my job. That's one thing I'm going to say. I love being here at [institution]. . . . And I, I'm here for students. That's what I'm here for." Sandie was also impassioned and harbored a deep understanding of the importance of affirming and validating her students as capable learners. This is demonstrated through her pedagogy; she explained:

I think the bigger thing I—that I teach them is confidence, is to believe in themselves, and that they can do this, and some of them have been told their whole lives they can't. Some of them have been told they're stupid. Some of them have been economically oppressed, whatever. Um, they get in this room where the first rule on the first day today is respect, and we're going to disagree, and we're going to have different opinions and different viewpoints and different lenses from which we've seen the world, but we're going to treat each other, um, and our communications with each other respectfully. . . . They've never had that. Nobody's ever said that to them.

Helping students build confidence was a recurring sentiment. Like Sandie, Ken has a similar orientation: "They've [students] been conditioned for years to think that they're not good at this [reading and composition]. And I help them rediscover it and look at it differently and maybe even learn to like it."

Listening to students and being reflective about her teaching practice was an important component of Harriet's pedagogy: "I want my students to think that I'm fair. So, I hope that I'm modeling good behavior, or ways of doing things, or thinking about things, you know, at the same time, I want to, I want to reflect on what they're saying to me and if they challenge me on something, I want to, I want to hear that, too."

Participants' pedagogies were a product of their backgrounds, teaching experiences, and dispositions as educators. I marveled at the examples provided about their student-centered, affirming, inclusive, empathic, caring, affect-conscious, and relational pedagogies. As mentioned prior, where they came from and who they are as educators informed and shaped how these faculty deployed these pedagogies.

## SUMMARY

This chapter was meant to foster in readers a sense of getting to know the faculty who were a part of this study. Their perceptions of and experiences with community college student mental health, which were shared during the interviews, provided a wellspring of information and insights. Yet prior to explicating what was shared about student mental health, it is critical to understand their career pathways, dispositions, and pedagogies, as these elements undergird and inform their perceptions, experiences, and insights.

The career pathways of these faculty are emblematic of what is typically shared within the literature. Community college faculty do not often intend to become community college faculty. But once in the role, many experience a deep enjoyment and love of teaching within the sector. They appreciate the teaching focus of the role and the sector; it is seen as a perk rather than a deterrent or shortcoming.

Faculty dispositions—their orientations to their work—certainly informed their behaviors within the role. These faculty loved teaching, and the diversity among their students was framed, largely, as being the best part of teaching. They gained both personal and professional fulfillment by facilitating student learning.

Their pedagogies—teaching approaches, methods, and strategies—were enveloped by student-centeredness, affirmation, inclusion, empathy, care, affect-consciousness, and being in relation to students. These characteristics of their pedagogies were affected by their dispositions and facilitated in them an ability to notice and accordingly engage with students who may be experiencing a mental health concern, which will be explained further in the next section.

It should be noted that the participants of the study self-selected, which means those who participated genuinely wanted to do so. Therefore, there is some level of self-selection bias inherent in the sample. Those who received the recruitment message and did not elect to participate may have dissimilar perceptions and experiences.

However, results generated through qualitative inquiry are not meant to be generalized to populations. Despite this, the information shared during the interviews is transferrable to other settings, and their insights are cogent. Much of what was shared is congruent with the literature, and the subtle deviations were opportunities for new insights and concomitant acumens on the topic of community college student mental health. The next chapter is focused on the ways faculty framed their students' assets as well as the obstacles they faced in pursuing their postsecondary educational goals.

## NOTES

1. See, for example, Danna Ethan and Erica J. Seidel, "On the Front Lines of Student Crisis: Urban Community College Professors' Experiences and Perceived Role in Handling Students in Distress," *College Student Affairs Journal* 31 no. 1 (Spring 2013): 15–26.

2. Amy L. Fugate and Marilyn J. Amey, "Career Stages of Community College Faculty: A Qualitative Analysis of Their Career Paths, Roles, and Development," *Community College Review* 28 no. 1 (Summer 2000): 1–22, https://doi.org/10.1177/009155210002800101.

3. Laura I. Rendón, "Validating Culturally Diverse Students: Toward a New Model of Learning and Student Development," *Innovative Higher Education* 19 no. 1 (September 1994): 33–51, https://doi.org/10.1007/BF01191156.

# Chapter 5

# Students' Assets and Obstacles

"I have in my drawer a 20-dollar bill. It stays there all the time because students sometimes need gas money . . . I can't just leave them [stranded]. You know, the mother comes out, and the grandma, in me. . . . I don't ask for it back, but they always do [give it back], so it replenishes for another student. But the barrier is money. They really don't have it."

–Camille

Faculty interviewed for this book talked a great deal about the range of assets and the obstacles students face in reaching their postsecondary education goals. Overwhelmingly, faculty cited resiliency as students' greatest asset. Resiliency is the capacity to endure difficult circumstances developed through previous experience of difficult circumstances. Tess encapsulated this well when she said:

I have students that have experienced very difficult things, which they are very often comfortable sharing. Things pertaining to like divorces, death of family, sexual assault, drug abuse, drug addiction, things like that. Um, but they're still showing up. And to me, that shows incredible resilience.

Carolyn mentioned something similar:

[T]hey've [students] done the hard thing. They've cleaned houses. They've waited tables, or whatever kind of work, and they said, "I want something better for me. I want something better for my kids. [Right now] I can't send my kids to college. I can't give my kids braces on their teeth. I want them to have a better life than I had."

While the diversity of the student body within the community college sector is a characteristic that makes it unique, many of these students have in common a wide range of marginalized identities (e.g., race, ethnicity,

93

nationality, citizen status, gender, sexuality, ability) and backgrounds. These identities and backgrounds are mediated by the disproportionate effects of socio-economic inequities, funding inequities within public K-12 schools, and endemic social forces. Some examples of these social forces include white supremacy and resultant systemic racism, American exceptionalism and resultant xenophobia, and heteronormativity and resultant homophobia. In the face of all this, students were described as *determined, courageous, hard-working,* and *survivors.*

Resiliency is a complicated concept, as it relies on the (past) presence of difficulty. Oftentimes, praising the resilient and promoting the development of resiliency takes precedence over the interrogation of why the difficult circumstance exists in the first place. For example, praising the resiliency of someone who has survived a domestic abuse situation is good, and helping someone in the process of domestic abuse survivorship is also good. At the same time, addressing the causes of domestic abuse is good, too. Yet the former is often the (sole) focus. And the latter is a cure.

If more focus were placed on changing the social context, like building more egalitarian cultural expectations about domestic relationships, increasing access to resources, removing obstacles, and ameliorating equity gaps, perhaps individuals would not need to be as resilient to survive the social context. The pain and suffering of enduring the difficulty could be spared.

Resiliency may come at a cost. Some of these costs may include post-traumatic stress, premature maturity, and unhealthy relationships with food. Building a world that does not require resilience is preferable to fostering resilience in individuals. Still, resiliency came through strongly within the interviews. Resiliency could also be framed as forms of capital,[1] community cultural wealth more specifically.[2] More on this (re)frame is forthcoming.

In a similarly overwhelming fashion, faculty said finances were students' most significant obstacle. For the most part, community colleges in the U.S. are committed to making higher education accessible for as many as possible. And for many individuals, the community college is a viable option because of its relative affordability.

Attending a community college is about a third of the cost of a public four-year institution.[3] As mentioned prior, many community college students come from poverty and/or are living in poverty. Even though the community college may seem affordable in comparative terms, it remains inaccessible for many even when considering the availability of grants and loans. For example, many prospective community college students may never have been exposed to the Free Application for Federal Student Aid. Availability is meaningless without access.

## ASSETS

Sandie used survivorship as an explanatory device when discussing student resilience. When difficult circumstances are all a student knows, that student may never have taken a moment to reflect on how resilient they have become, which can be empowering—for that student as well as others. She said:

> I think they [students] have survived, a lot of them, so much garbage that playing the game of getting through college is nothing [in comparison]. Once they figure it out, once they understand you gotta show up, you gotta do the work, you gotta be respectful to your professors, they can do that. I mean, some of them have maneuvered abusive relationships. Some of them have come from, um, alcoholic parents. Some of them are struggling with drugs and alcohol themselves. You know, in the middle of that. If you can kick those things, you can live through those things, you can get through college algebra. Somebody just needs to say that to them, because all their lives they've heard "college" and pictured smart people, and never identified themselves as that person, and so I think once you can light that fire, they're on fire, and they're amazing because they warm the people around them. Other people see that spark. Other people are attracted to that. Other people want to take a ride with that because they see it moving forward. It's just lighting it, which sometimes is really hard to do when they're still in a, such a dark place sometimes.

Like Sandie, Phoebe, who taught legal studies, told a story about a student whose husband inundated her with negative sentiments for *a year*, saying she was not smart enough to be a paralegal. That difficult context, coupled with concerted engagement with the program and support from Phoebe, fostered resiliency within the student. It also created a context in which the student could question and eventually reject the messaging from her husband. Within the classroom, the student's skills, ability, and work ethic were recognized and valued. This helped her realize and believe she *was* smart enough to be a paralegal. About this student, Phoebe said:

> They really, really respond, and hear you when you say, "You, you're really doing it." . . . [Student] came down, she wanted me to go over her motion for preliminary objection, which is due tomorrow. I said, "This is as good as any lawyer's motion."

Phoebe's comments also suggest that resiliency can provide students with the tools necessary to believe in change and embrace a growth mindset.[4] Embodying a growth mindset means acting in accordance with the belief that abilities can be developed. Growth mindset contrasts with a fixed mindset, which translates into acting in accordance with the belief that abilities are fixed traits. Phoebe explained how a growth mindset can help students realize the possibility of a new kind of life context. About this, Phoebe said:

> They know when they are improving, and it allows them to see that you can change. And, you can be better, and you're not going to be stuck, um, just because you always were some way. And, I think that's kind of one of the hardest things about getting out of any bad place, is thinking you can't change, or because people all around you are saying that [you can't change].

She continued that when students see that they are improving and begin to develop a growth mindset, that can end up being "their biggest strength."

Similarly, Joy offered many stories about how students in her program (human services) are very motivated and have changed their lives. This could be seen as what Yosso termed aspirational capital.[5] Joy said some students are "incredibly persistent and strong." She continued:

> They have not given up, and they keep coming back until they get it [a credential]. And, so, that's one of the things that always amazes me. I mean, I've had students who have literally started out on the street in a shelter and have managed to go from there to having a bachelor or a master's degree. And I can go out into the community and see them working now. . . . Those people are, are inspirational.

Rose offered similar commentary: "So many students I met here are so resilient. You know, they, they are so determined to succeed. And frequently it's some of the ones who have the most responsibilities." Those responsibilities range from juggling elder care, parenting, and holding several jobs, not to mention completing college coursework.

In another example of a student's embodiment of resiliency, Stephanie shared that she had a student who started falling behind in her class, and when she reached out to her to see how she was doing and check in, the student shared she had been going through some tough times. She confided in Stephanie that she had been homeless, living in her car with her two children for several months. As a former heroin addict, she did not want to go to the shelters or stay with a family member who offered her space, because she knew she would be exposed to drugs at both places.

Stephanie was floored. She told her: "Are you sure you can be in school when you don't even have a roof over your head? And you're trying to focus on these writing silly papers in a class and yet, you don't have a roof over your head." To Stephanie's amazement, her student persisted. "She proved me wrong," Stephanie shared. "She got through the semester with a B in my class, and I'm pretty sure she got through all of her other classes." No doubt, dealing with dire life circumstances and demonstrating resilience was a core strength that community college faculty identified as emblematic of their students.

## OBSTACLES

Faculty described the many obstacles their students must face in the ongoing pursuit of their educational goals. While some mentioned academic or cognitive challenges, such as a lack of what might be considered college-level writing skills, most of the obstacles referenced had nothing to do with academics. In fact, most community college student attrition can be attributed to *everything but* academic ability or achievement.

The most mentioned challenge was financial. This is significant. Financial stress is a *major* contributor to mental health problems among community college students.[6] Many resultant challenges stemmed from this one pernicious challenge, including living in poverty, homelessness and housing insecurity, food insecurity, access to childcare, and unreliable transportation.

Many of these resultant challenges are mental health correlates. For example, community college students with basic needs insecurity are more likely to suffer from mental health issues than their needs-secure peers.[7] Some of these obstacles may seem like a temporary inconvenience, but Rebecca, for example, explained how "those [lack of funds for car repair] are the kinds of things that can destroy a student's semester, especially if they live a distance away."

Again, for those with the privilege of financial security, something such as caring for a sick child who was sent home from school, dealing with a flat tire, or missing the bus may seem like a minor setback, a blip in the day, or a small inconvenience. However, for many community college students, things like this can be disastrous.

Justin explained that many students are "just one flat tire away" from disaster. If they cannot get to campus or if they cannot get all the books or supplies they need, their success in college will suffer. If they cannot get to work because of transportation issues, they can't receive a paycheck, and that means they can't pay their living expenses, let alone tuition for courses they are taking. As he put it, any sort of transportation issue will lead to major financial issues, and that "creates difficulties in their lives, which translate and affect their function in the classroom."

Sandie explained how her relational pedagogy created an environment wherein students felt comfortable asking her for help regarding some of these obstacles that not only impeded pursuit of their educational goals, but also created difficulties for their wellbeing and their family's wellbeing. She said:

I've had students come to me because they missed class because they were living in a one-bedroom [in] basically a condemned building, and they had bedbugs, and it was winter, [and they had] no blanket. They didn't know . . . what to do, "What do we do with our blankets and our sheets? I'm taking care of my mom." You know, and this is a student who's not trying to create favor with me. This is a student who I've built this relationship with over the semester and came to me and said, "I'm really embarrassed to ask anybody else for help. What do I do?"

Joy's comments spoke to the interconnected and related nature of the barriers students faced, starting with not having enough income. She said:

We have students coming in here with very limited resources sometimes. . . . students who are really trying to get ahead and really wanna be here and really wanna work hard, but they're working against a lot of barriers at home. You know, they don't have enough income. . . . I've had students who were on the street homeless. I've had students with significant mental health problems. I've had students, um, who, you know, were still living at home but that family situation wasn't too good. I've had students who were in relationships that made me really worried at times. Like, is this person, is this going to turn into a domestic violence situation?

She worried about her students having "so much going on" in their lives. Financial crises, family members with terminal illnesses, losing loved ones, homelessness, abuse and trauma, not to mention mental health challenges and going to college—it all seemed like too much for her students to handle.

One faculty member, Carolyn, used the phrase "chaotic lives" to summarize the challenges her students faced. She said for some of her students, they "have chaotic lives. Many of them. I mean, really chaotic." She mentioned that a big barrier was money, or lack thereof. She described how students often prioritized work instead of college—and for good reason. Some may need to maintain full-time work to provide health insurance for their family.

On the one hand, this can be seen as a rational choice, but on the other hand, it can be seen as a barrier to academic success. Carolyn continued: "they get financial aid . . . but they usually have to work as well, and sometimes they have to work more hours, and then the boss wants them to work overtime, and then they don't get to class." Geraldine used an apt metaphor to explain students having chaotic lives, which can result in attrition. She said:

They drop out of class because they cannot manage the balance between their work and between their school, and between their kids, and between, they can't, they cannot, keep all their balls in the air.

Geraldine reflected on how conflicted this made her feel as a faculty member who cared about her students and also wanted to "keep the integrity of the curriculum." She shared "that's what really makes me, not lose sleep, but that's what really concerns me." These quotes reflect how students' lives are almost always "chaotic" when financial resources are sparse and difficult decisions must be made as a result.

On top of financial difficulties, Sophie mentioned students do not always have strong support systems in place. She explained:

> I feel like . . . whereas I might get sick, and I have a lot of support from family and friends. And I think that's what's lacking a lot in these students: they don't have a big support system.

She explained that she's had students who had to miss a couple classes in a row because their children were sick. There are "no alternatives" for her students because of their lack of a support system. It can be very difficult. She explained, "When we hit this bump, what now? How do we pick ourselves up and keep going?" While Sophie's perspective is certainly earnest, not having support systems in place may also be a proxy for financial constraints. Support systems can be bought. For example, childcare, eldercare, grocery delivery, and transportation can be purchased if you have the money. So, again, it really comes down to finances.

There was some mention of students' educational and cultural backgrounds, which were framed as deficits within the community college context. For example, some faculty mentioned first-generation college students were alienated or ostracized from their families for pursuing college. Some mentioned that because many Hispanic and/or Latinx/a/o students' families prioritize family and community above all else, students are unable to focus on or prioritize college-related commitments. In one example, a student missed class to pick up his nephew from school. In another, a student spent two weeks in Puerto Rico for a relative's funeral, which meant not attending classes.

This perspective frames students as not being *college-ready* or not having the *cultural capital* to understand college culture.[8] It disregards the notion that the college may not be *student-ready*.[9] It also disregards the cultural wealth contained in these students' *familial capital*.[10] That said, framing students' cultural backgrounds as having deficits should be interrogated and contested.

Because of their open access imperative community colleges *must* work with the students they have. Rather than resisting this reality, it must be embraced. For some, this represents a paradigm shift regarding how higher education is conceptualized. Rather than expecting students to be college-ready, community colleges must (aspire to) be student-ready. This includes "reframing the student success conversation from one of precollege characteristics and student deficits to one of student assets and institutional opportunity, leadership, and accountability."[11]

Being a student-ready college can be controlled by community college personnel, whereas community college personnel cannot control whether students are college-ready. In fact, expecting incoming students to be college-ready is antithetical to open-door admissions policies and the access mission of the nation's community colleges. Aspiring toward student-readiness is an agentic position for community colleges. Student-readiness highlights student assets and institutional openness and dexterity. College-readiness highlights student deficits and institutional stubbornness and stagnation.

According to Yosso, community cultural wealth (CCW) is a critical race critique of cultural capital.[12] CCW highlights the knowledges and skills of marginalized communities of color. The unique forms of cultural capital present within these communities often goes unrecognized and undervalued. Forms of capital recognized and affirmed through this lens include aspirational, navigational, social, linguistic, familial, and resistant. Yosso argued that "the main goals of identifying and documenting cultural wealth are to transform education and empower People of Color to utilize assets already abundant in their communities."[13]

As noted in the example above, some participants mentioned Hispanic and/or Latinx/a/o students' community- and family-focused culture (e.g., familial capital) and framed it as a deficit. This framing signals to Hispanic and/or Latinx/a/o that their culture is a detriment to their success. This is problematic.

These students' cultural backgrounds should be framed as a form of cultural wealth (i.e., familial capital)—one that institutions should understand, embrace, and be *ready for*. Implementing flexibly attendance policies is one example. Institutional leaders should combine notions of student-readiness with the concept of CCW to promote student success rather than impose barriers to it.

## Obstacles as Indicators of Institutional and Systemic Issues

Institutional barriers such as individual- and system-level errors with placement testing and developmental education were also mentioned. For example, Suzie told the story of an African American woman who tested into college-level English but was placed into remedial reading and writing. If Suzie had not checked her scores and moved her, this student would have wasted a lot of time and money.

Issues and inequities concerning developmental education have long been in play within the community college policy and research landscape. The situation Suzie described is not uncommon. As part of the completion agenda,[14] many states and individual institutions have pursued major developmental reforms. Yet these issues persist.

That faculty noted financial issues as the number one obstacle students face in their pursuit of higher education is unsurprising. It highlights several systemic issues that have resulted in inequitable student access to and success within higher education. These issues include capitalism and its relationship to socio-economic stratification, neoliberalism and its relationship to viewing higher education as a private good, and white supremacy and its relationship to higher education culture and funding. It is easy to frame barriers as student deficits, then highlight those deficits as the big reasons why students are not successful. But systemic forces like those mentioned above are the real culprit.

For example, income levels are highly stratified within the United States,[15] which largely operates under a capitalist economic model. Access to certain college types is influenced by parental income. Children of parents in the top one percent of the income distribution in the United States are 77 times more likely to attend an elite institution as compared to children of parents who are in the fifth quintile of the income distribution. At the same time, conditional on the college they attend, students from low- and high-income backgrounds had comparable earning outcomes. In other words, the students from low-income backgrounds at an elite institution belonged there.[16]

Neoliberalism prizes individualism, privatization, and free markets. Neoliberal forces have framed higher education as an exclusively private good. This vantage point highlights the private benefits of higher education (e.g., earning potential) but often renders invisible the public ones (e.g., civic engagement, decreased recidivism). As a result, many states have disinvested in higher education over time.[17] This is dangerous because evidence suggests increased state support for higher education is directly tied to student success.[18] As a result, many college students are paying the price.[19]

Finally, white supremacy is another force endemic to United States society, of which higher education is a part. We are constantly living within the cumulative result of history. As an example, there is a significant gap in white and Black wealth, which is a result of slavery, Jim Crow-era laws, and ongoing racial inequities.[20] Moreover, many students of color who attend predominantly white institutions *still* feel like guests in another's home.[21] At the same time, many minority-serving institutions such as historically Black colleges and universities and tribal colleges, some of which are two-year institutions, are inequitably funded.[22]

Here is the point: the obstacles community college students face are not the result of individual student failure(s). Instead, they are indicators of institutional and systemic issues. The students are not the problem. The problems reside within institutions and the systems in which those institutions are enmeshed. Using an asset-based and ecological view of community college students and their mental health is a key step in understanding and addressing this issue. These ideas are expanded in the final section of the book.

## SUMMARY

Faculty in this study described the many assets their students possessed, which were propelling forces in those students' ability to persist toward their postsecondary educational goals. On the other hand, faculty also articulated the barriers students faced along the way. Resiliency was the most prevalent asset. Students were seen as survivors. And financial challenges stemming from systemic issues were the most prevalent obstacle. This is vital to understanding community college student mental health because money-related stress is a source of mental health issues and concerns among students.[23]

Within this section of the book, I outlined information gleaned from interviews with community college faculty regarding their career pathways, pedagogies, dispositions, and what they viewed as their students' most salient assets and obstacles. This context is helpful in building a full picture of how these faculty perceive and experience their students' mental health, which is the focus of the following section.

## NOTES

1. Pierre Bourdieu, "The Forms of Capital," in *Handbook of Theory and Research for the Sociology of Education,* ed. John Richardson (Westport, CT: Greenwood. 1986): 241–258.

2. Tara J. Yosso, "Whose Culture Has Capital? A Critical Race Theory of Community Cultural Wealth," *Race Ethnicity and Education* 8 no. 1 (2005): 69–91. https://doi.org/10.1080/1361332052000341006.

3. American Association of Community Colleges (AACC), "Fast Facts 2022," Research Trends, revised May 11, 2022, https://www.aacc.nche.edu/research-trends/fast-facts/.

4. Carol S. Dweck, *Mindset: The New Psychology of Success* (New York: Ballantine, 2006).

5. Yosso, "Whose Culture Has Capital?"

6. Sarah Ketchen Lipson et al., "Mental Health Conditions Among Community College Students: A National Study of Prevalence and Use of Treatment Services,"

*Psychiatric Services* 72, no. 10 (October 2021): 1126–1133, https://doi.org/10.1176/appi.ps.202000437.

7. Katherine M. Broton, Milad Mohebali, and Mitchell D. Lingo, "Basic Needs Insecurity and Mental Health: Community College Students' Dual Challenges and Use of Social Support," *Community College Review* 50, no. 4 (2022): 456–482.

8. Bourdieu, "The Forms of Capital."

9. Tia Brown McNair et al., *Becoming a Student-Ready College: A New Culture of Leadership for Student Success,* 2nd ed. (Hoboken, NJ: Jossey-Bass, 2022).

10. Yosso, "Whose Culture Has Capital?"

11. Brown McNair, *Becoming a Student-Ready College.*

12. Yosso, "Whose Culture Has Capital?"

13. Yosso, "Whose Culture Has Capital?" 82.

14. Christopher Baldwin, *The Completion Agenda in Community Colleges: What It Is, Why It Matters, and Where It's Going* (Lanham, MD: Rowman & Littlefield, 2017).

15. Emily A. Shrider et al., *U.S. Census Bureau Current Population Reports P60-273, Income and Poverty in the United States: 2020* (Washington, DC: U.S. Government Publishing Office, September 2021), https://www.census.gov/content/dam/Census/library/publications/2021/demo/p60-273.pdf.

16. Raj Chetty et al., "Mobility Report Cards: The Role of Colleges in Intergenerational Mobility," NBER Working Paper No. 23618, Revised Version, Opportunity Insights, Harvard University, Cambridge, MA, December 2017, https://opportunityinsights.org/paper/mobilityreportcards/; Raj Chetty et al., "Mobility Report Cards: The Role of Colleges in Intergenerational Mobility," Opportunity Insights, Harvard University, Cambridge, MA, July 2017, https://opportunityinsights.org/wp-content/uploads/2018/03/coll_mrc_paper.pdf; Raj Chetty et al., "Income Segregation and Intergenerational Mobility Across Colleges in the United States," *Quarterly Journal of Economics* 135, no. 3 (August 2020): 1567–1633.

17. Richard J. Greenfield and Ermasova Natalia, "Disinvestment in Higher Education and its Impact on Society: Case of Illinois Universities, *Public Education Review* (August 2022), https://doi.org/10.1007/s11115-022-00649-2.

18. Kristen Cummings et al., *Investigating the Impacts of Higher Education Appropriations and Financial Aid,* State Higher Education Executive Officers Association, May 2021, https://sheeo.org/wp-content/uploads/2021/05/SHEEO_ImpactAppropationsFinancialAid.pdf.

19. Sara Goldbrick-Rab, *Paying the Price* (Chicago: University of Chicago Press, 2016).

20. Melvin Oliver and Thomas M. Shapiro, eds., *Black Wealth/White Wealth: A New Perspective on Racial Inequality,* 2nd ed. (New York: Routledge, 2006).

21. Caroline Sotello Viernes Turner, "Guests in Someone Else's House: Students of Color," *The Review of Higher Education* 17, no. 4 (Summer 1994): 335–370. https://muse.jhu.edu/article/644635/pdf.

22. Adam Harris, *The State Must Provide: The Definitive History of Racial Inequality in American Higher Education* (New York: HarperColllins, 2022).

23. Ketchen Lipson et al., "Mental Health Conditions."

# PART III

# The Discussions

This section outlines the various dimensions of the discussions with faculty specifically regarding their students' mental health. Chapter 6 is focused on faculty emotional labor. Through the interviews, it became clear emotional labor was a prerequisite for faculty to perceive or notice the affective components of their students' educational lives. It was the gateway through which they were able to perceive, experience, and grow understandings of their students' mental health.

Chapter 7 is focused on the importance of rejecting monolithic thinking regarding community college students who have or may have mental health concerns or issues. Within this chapter a perceptual typology of students is presented, which was built, *literally*, from the interview data. This typology, or model, can be a helpful framework, but it should not be viewed as an absolute.

Chapter 8 focuses on how faculty navigated institutional structures and systems within the context of student mental health. Referral to counseling and making behavioral intervention team (BIT) reports were points of discussion throughout the interviews.

Finally, chapter 9 features faculty advice for other faculty. Through the interviews, it was clear the participants in this study were good at their jobs. Based on what they have learned along the way, they shared invaluable insights on what advice they would give new faculty related to student mental health. Much of what is contained in this chapter is based on participants' experiences and learning through trial and error.

# Chapter 6

# Doing Emotional Labor

"I think the opportunity is there to make the biggest difference.... They're [students] at junctures in their lives.... and I want to be part of that juncture in their lives."

–Carolyn

As highlighted prior, faculty can play an important role in the educational lives of students, and this goes beyond the physical, cognitive, and intellectual aspects of faculty work. As Pam stated, "[t]he students' number one resource is the faculty." Being a resource for students often involves emotional labor.

Emotional labor was first coined by Arlie Hochschild in 1983.[1] In her original conception, the term was defined as being paid to feel the feelings appropriate for doing a certain job. The oft-cited example is the work of flight attendants who are paid to be polite and friendly in the face of a sometimes stressful work environment. Being cognizant of, regulating, and managing one's own emotions along with others' is necessary to do the job well. Emotional labor is embedded in work that involves other people.[2] Examples of emotional labor include listening, talking, empathizing, and assessing personalities.

Since the term's inception, it has been tinkered with and expanded by scholars and within popular culture.[3] It has gained traction within the field of higher education and been applied to faculty work, generating important insights.[4]

Within the context of this study, emotional labor is conceived of as the work faculty do to create, understand, manage, and regulate their own feelings and the feelings of their students within educational (e.g., classrooms, LMS course sites) and education-adjacent (e.g., email, physical office space) contexts. There was a clear connection between faculty doing emotional labor and having perceptions of and experiences with community college students' mental health. It was a prerequisite, in fact.

As was evident in the previous section, faculty dispositions and pedagogies suggested they fostered relationships with students, which were characterized by *seeing* and talking with students, expressing empathy, and offering care. They *knew* their students. Their labor was not just cognitive or intellectual. Their labor was very often emotional—centered on feelings—and their pedagogies were affect-conscious rather than affect-evasive. Affect consciousness among these faculty meant being aware of and in tune with the affective elements of oneself as an educator, the learning space, and the learners in the learning space.

Their dispositions laid the foundation for their pedagogical ontologies—ways of *being* as faculty members. From these ontological positions, they did not exclusively teach developmental English, sonography, nursing, art history, or respiratory therapy, they taught *community college students*. This (re)framing was part of fore-fronting their students rather than the subjects to be taught, which meant the affective components of learning and the learning environment were just as if not more important than the cognitive-intellectual components.

Here, Kucirka's work warrants highlighting.[5] She carried out a grounded theory study, which included interviews with 13 nursing faculty about their interactions with nursing students with mental health issues within a four-year institution context. As a result, she created a substantive theory about these interactions. The theory includes a four-phase process: noticing, responding, experiencing, and reflecting.

Overall, the data collected through my study corroborate Kucirka's theory—with one key exception: noticing comes from a context, and that context is an affect-conscious pedagogical ontology that requires emotional labor.[6] I would, therefore, expand her theory to five phases: doing emotional labor, noticing, responding, experiencing, and reflecting.

Furthermore, community college faculty may be able to provide better insights on their students' mental health than their faculty counterparts at four-year institutions. Teaching is the main and most time-consuming task of most community college faculty. In contrast, some faculty at four-year institutions do not teach at all. Kucirka noted that her participants may have been "too stressed themselves to recognize and acknowledge student stress" because of their "heavy workloads, pressure to maintain scholarship and actively participate in . . . committees."[7]

While full-time community college faculty may have other duties that compete with teaching, many of those duties involve working with students in other capacities (e.g., advising). On the other hand, most adjunct faculty are only contracted to teach, so most of their work at the institution is relegated to the classroom. It may be that most community college faculty know their students better than most faculty at four-year institutions as a function of how their time is spent—*with students.*

## PROGRAM MEDIATED EMOTIONAL LABOR

Sometimes, the affective and the cognitive-intellectual components of learning are tightly knit together to the point of being inextricable. Ken provided an example of how sometimes students have clinical experiences that may be traumatic. Doing emotional labor on behalf of students in these situations can be especially difficult. He told the following story:

> I've only ever had to really do it one time, but we had students at [a] clinical site, and they went to a trauma that was a horrific trauma of a person who had gotten caught in live electrical wires. And was a teenager, was burnt, the whole nine yards. Instructor calls me, he says, 'Hey, I just want you to know this is what's going on that what you're seeing on the news and—and I said, "Okay. Have you done a debrief with the students?" "Yes." [response] And we pulled each one of them in individually. And, you know, explain to them this is probably one of the most horrific things you're ever going to see, and you need to understand that this person is going to die even though they took him to the burn center. Here's what's going to happen, and it happened exactly as I told them it was gonna. But I'm like, "Here's what's going to happen, and he is going to die regardless, but you are never going to get that smell or that image out of your mind. You need to understand, if you start exhibiting any signs or symptoms [related to mental health concerns in response to the trauma], somebody mentions it to you, we see it or you see it in yourself, you must notify me immediately. We have people that you can talk to that you can, you know, can help you with that."

As is evident within this quotation, the affective and the cognitive-intellectual components of learning within this specific clinical incident are so tightly knit they are nearly indistinguishable.

In addition, it should be noted that some program cultures, especially highly selective and cohort-based programs, may have relational elements built into them. For example, warm and inclusive policy language in syllabi, curricula focused on high-quality patient care, long laboratory hours spent together, and having similar educational and career goals can facilitate a relational culture among students and faculty. Nurturing these relational program elements requires emotional labor.

That faculty engage in emotional labor, therefore, may be an expectation within some programs and part of the faculty socialization process. Ken explained that when he "became the [respiratory therapy] program director, we changed tones. And I have very much gone a little bit more with the kinder gentler [language]." This language change is an example of emotional labor.

Christina alluded to the relational nature of the sonography program:

> We [faculty and students in the program] have a very close relationship. And so, you do. You get . . . you get attached to the students, you kind of feel like their mom, and . . . you kind of watch out for them. . . . It is a totally different relationship than a professor would [who] might have them for psychology one semester, and that's all they see them for, you know what I mean?

Because students within this program spend so much time together and in close proximity to their faculty, close relationships emerge as a result. This simply does not happen within other programs, as Christina mentioned.

## KNOWING STUDENTS THROUGH EMOTIONAL LABOR

Consider again that the faculty who volunteered to participate in this study self-selected. They willingly responded to the open call for participants sent to the entire faculty population at the institution. That said, it cannot be assumed the participants are representative of the population. Therefore, it is highly likely that not all faculty engage in emotional labor and execute their pedagogies and ontologies in the ways explained here. Camille expressed this well:

> You've got to know your students. See that's the—some people [faculty] don't take time to get to know them [students] . . . How do you know if they're having a bad affect, if you have no idea who they really are? Who they normally are? Like if I can't look at my student and know their name, the color of their eyes, it means I never look at them.

The sentiments within this interview excerpt are rich with insights into Camille's teaching disposition and pedagogical approaches, both of which are imbued with emotional labor and affect consciousness. Again, affect consciousness is noticing the affective, or the feeling and emotional, elements of the learning environment and the students who are a part of that environment.

And there is evidence here to suggest that some faculty do not engage in the labor necessary to know students, which will be expanded upon later in this chapter. As she highlighted, if there is no consciousness of who students *are*, then there can be no perception of *changes* in who students are, which will later be explained as an important part of noticing signs of mental health issues.

Jody emphasized that "you don't really know what's going on [with a student] until you take the time to really get to know a student." Not only does this knowing take time, it also requires a pedagogical approach that emphasizes building rapport and a willingness to do emotional labor.

## Empathy and Solidarity as Emotional Labor

Camille proudly told a story about one of her students, whom she calls her "success story." Kimberly (a pseudonym) is a Black female student who moved from the noncredit workforce area to the credit area within Early Childhood Education. Had Camille not taken the time to really get to know Kimberly and her life circumstances, Kimberly's trajectory through college could have played out much differently.

One of Camille's faculty colleagues lamented and complained to her one day that Kimberly fell asleep in her class. In response, Camille told her "Let her sleep. Because, you know, she's up all night with her kids at the hospital." It was apparent to Camille that her colleague did not realize all that Kimberly was trying to juggle in addition to college. Camille proudly reported that Kimberly graduated from the program:

> I think she's going to be our student of the year. And it took a lot for her to finish. Well look at her family situation. And she's also [in addition to having children with sickle cell anemia] raising her grandchildren. Because I have a close relative in jail—so I frequent prisons, and she . . . she has family in jail. So we compare jail stories. . . . but I'm telling you, she is my success story.

This quote demonstrates that Camille is the type of faculty member who not only gets to know her students' life circumstances, but she also shares her own life circumstances to build connection and rapport and cultivate empathy and solidarity with them.

Sandie described how she tries to normalize help-seeking behavior among her students *and* make it easier for them. She explained:

> I don't think it's helpful for people in crisis to say, "Here's someone that will help you," because I've been in crisis, and I think when you're in it, sometimes it's all you can do to just be upright, much less track down help . . . And the fact that they've made the effort to come to me to get the help—that's the effort. It's now my responsibility to at least attempt to procure that help for them.

She also described how she shares her own experiences to build emotional connection with students and further normalize seeking mental health support. She shared, "I think with students it helps to, instead of just saying, 'You need therapy.' Sometimes it helps to personalize it by saying, 'Well, you're like me, and I've had therapy, and look, I, you don't think [any less of me].'" Here again, expressing empathy and solidarity is a form of faculty emotional labor.

This is not to say referrals to on-campus support personnel are inappropriate; Camille is simply making a note about timing, tone, and the positive effect of getting to know your students on a personal and emotional level.

## AFFIRMING AND VALIDATING
## AS EMOTIONAL LABOR

Using affirmation to communicate to students the validity of their experiences, feelings, identities, and/or personhoods was another form of emotional labor among faculty. Sandie told the following story about a trans man in one of her classes:

> I had a student who was transitioning who said to me about the third week, "Stop calling me Susan. I want you to call me Chris. I identify as Chris. I know you don't understand it, but this is who I am, and I hope to be making a journey on this progress that I started a few months ago." Um, I was able to say, "You know what? Let's connect you with these people who will tell you how you fill out the paperwork here so you show up on my roll sheet as Chris, not Susan." . . . And I think prior to that he felt very marginalized. He'd been disowned by his mother. It's gonna make me cry. Um, he had been disowned by his mother for transitioning. He was sort of in this . . . gray space of, I don't know where I fit into the world, and I think that coming here and finding somebody—me—who was supportive of what he was doing and honored that, and then not only honored that, was able to say, "Look, let's help. Let me help you."

Needless to say, emotional labor is hard emotional work. As this quote shows, Sandie got emotional reflecting on this student and the impact she had on him, and the impact he had on her.

Justin, an adjunct who taught sociology, told a beautiful story about a former student who was in recovery and formerly incarcerated. This story showcases the many benefits of engaging in emotional labor for students. Justin recounted a story about a student from several years ago. At the time, the student was living in a men's shelter while taking classes.

He talked about how the student "came in . . . and he was so soft spoken, so shy, and so unsure of himself, that it was painful to watch him go through the process." In time, the student "was floundering, and he came to me after class one night, and . . . said 'I guess, I just don't, I just don't think I fit in here. I just don't think I, this is for me.'" Justin talked with the student for a long time. He asked the student "what would happen that would make you feel like you fit in?"

Justin affirmed this student and validated his experiences, both in and outside the classroom, and engaged in conversation with him. He continued:

> He says "I just have this feeling, I just don't belong here, you know?" And I, I told him, I said . . . we had a paper due the next week. I said "I want to see your paper. Don't give up yet . . . I want you to write a paper. I want you to do the best you can; I want you to write the paper. I don't want you to care about grammar and spelling. I mean I want that [paper] to be as good as you can make it, but . . . don't give up on yourself. I want to read it, and I want to, I want to sit down and talk to you about it." And when I read it I, it was, like, this guy has some of the best insights in the class. He doesn't really know how to express them very well, but when you, when you really . . . start breaking it down, it was like okay, this guy kind of gets clients . . . and situations. Well anyway, I use him now every semester as a presenter for the class at [the men's shelter], okay? And, he can stand now, in front of my class, for an hour and a half and give an awesome presentation on the, and it is a fantastic program, that they have up there, um, but the thought of him doing that fifteen years ago was so foreign to everybody around him that he, there's just absolutely no way that could have been real, you know, for him. . . . [name] and I are friends now, you know what I mean? It's that kind of thing where he just had to be convinced "you're okay here. You, you're gonna make it, you're gonna be okay."

Justin listened, affirmed the student's situation, and offered encouragement. He also embodied and deployed a deep and unwavering commitment to this student's success. His use of I-statements (e.g., "I want you to do the best you can.") was powerful in this story—and likely to the student. These acts of emotional labor cultivated in the student a sense of belonging, which was originally lacking.

## Listening as Affirmation and Validation

Interviews suggested that, from the faculty member's standpoint, engaging in emotional labor may be a prerequisite for noticing that a student is exhibiting symptoms of stress or mental health issues. The behaviors that faculty engaged in after noticing those symptoms may also involve emotional labor, such as asking questions and listening, as well as efforts to tweak and sharpen pedagogies informed by affect consciousness. Tess explained that if she had a student she thought might be exhibiting symptoms of a mental health issue, she would proceed in a certain emotionally attuned way:

I would just kind of pull the student aside or ask them to see me during office hours, and kind of ask them about how things are going. "What's going on? What, you know, tell me about you as a student, what's happening here."

When Tess has taken that approach before, she has had two or three students share with her that they were struggling with anxiety or depression. In response, she would, as she put it, "kind of explore with them" about what that meant. She would listen and ask if there was anything she could "do differently in the classroom" to help them and support them.

Listening to students is implicit in Tess's approach and a hallmark of many participants in the study. As will be discussed later in the book, while it is critical for faculty to facilitate student referrals to resources both on- and off-campus (e.g., counseling center, food pantry), listening to a student requires no professional training, license, or credential in mental health, though that certainly helps.

Eve said in plain terms: "for many students, they just need somebody to listen to them." Rose provided examples of how she opens herself to listening to students; she tells them:

"If you want to tell me what's going on, please feel free, I'd be more than happy to listen." or, "Just tell me as much information as you feel comfortable telling me," all of that kind of stuff. And they'll tell me some extremely difficult things.

Listening is a gift faculty can give to students, but it is laborious. Eve also mentioned that there are limits to what one faculty member can do for a student, and the work of teaching a full-time teaching load can be overwhelming in and of itself.

Like Eve, Suzie said "Basically, I do a lot of listening. . . . Sometimes they [students] just need someone to listen." And while Suzie noted listening to students and carrying out emotional labor, she also said "I'm also, you know, tough, I think." She shared that she's aware of her limits: "I can't save everybody, you know?"

Martin told a story wherein the importance of tone within conversation with students really mattered. Attentiveness to these sorts of communicative details was prevalent among the faculty. Many community college students enter the space after having negative and damaging experiences with teachers and others inside educational spaces such as K-12 schools and other institutions of higher education.

The intentionality of community college faculty approaches to communication with students is another example of emotional labor. Martin said:

[T]his young Hispanic man was leaving the class one day and he stopped, and he turned around and he said, "Mr. [last name], do you realize you're the first teacher I've ever had to talk *with* me, and *not* down to me?" And so, through that interaction, I think they realized that I really am their champion, and I'm here to help them and I mean I, I'll give them my cell phone number. I'll meet them after hours. I'll do whatever I can to help them succeed. And I think that they know that's sincere.

Simply listening to students can be affirming and validating to them, and the faculty participants within this study took that seriously. While listening can be laborious, it does not require a specific license or credential. Listening to students does, however, require a willingness and a decision to do so. And as the next section describes, these kinds of decisions are often gendered.

## EMOTIONAL LABOR AS GENDERED

Bellas outlined the gender-based nature of emotional labor among university faculty across four work domains of the professoriate: research, teaching, service, and administration.[8] She noted that women faculty spend more time on teaching and service than they do on research and administration. In addition, she argued that teaching and service work are emotionally laborious, undervalued, and largely invisible.

In contrast, she stated that men faculty spend more time on research and administration than they do on teaching and service. These endeavors, she argued, involve some level of emotional labor, but that labor is overshadowed by notions that research and administrative work require intellectual, strategic, and technical labor, which is more highly valued, visible, and incentivized, rewarded, and compensated, at least across four-year universities. While situated within the four-year sector, glimmers of Bellas's assertions were evident within the present study's data.[9]

Affect-conscious pedagogies frame students as emotional beings who have feelings and who emote. When students' emotional selves are affirmed and validated, they may view being in communication with faculty as a safe space for feelings to exist and manifest and to be expressed. Phoebe said:

I used to share an office with a [male colleague] and he used to make fun of me, because he said, "All your students come in and just cry." [laughing] . . . Yeah, it was a safe place. . . . Um. And it seemed like everybody had something.

In the above excerpt, it is interesting to hear Phoebe describe her male colleague as using humor to tease her about being an emotionally available faculty member with whom students felt safe to share their feelings. The emotional labor of faculty has long been invisible, unrewarded, considered unserious, and framed as in opposition to intellectual labor. Yet, it was a critical pillar within the work of these faculty members.

Within this study and elsewhere, emotional labor is characterized as gendered. Recall that 86 percent of the participants of this study identified as women and all self-selected. Emotional labor is often associated with women, and there was some evidence to suggest that the participants of this study viewed men as doing less emotional labor. Suzie said:

> I think I am somebody who is unable to not ask a student if there's something wrong. Um, and that, I think, means that I end up in a lot more of these sorts of conversations [about mental health]. And I think a lot of people maybe have more sense. I know I have a male faculty member, say, to say to me, he doesn't do emotional lifting. And I thought, "That must be very nice."

Implied here is that Suzie's pedagogic ontology compels her to engage in emotional labor, which, even in jest, she seems to connect to *not* being sensible. And her more sensible (i.e., rational) man colleague is relieved of doing this type of work, and she envies him. There is some evidence to suggest women and transgender and nonbinary faculty act more frequently as referral agents regarding student mental health concerns than men.[10]

While all the men in this study engaged in significant emotional labor, the general sense was that women do this work more. This requires further interrogation. There may be other mediating factors as well, as evidenced elsewhere, such as experience, race, subject area, and experience.[11]

## BOUNDARIES AND CAPACITIES

While engaging in emotional labor was an important facet of these faculty members' work, especially considering student mental health, taking care of oneself is also vital. Listening comes at a cost. Listening takes time. Faculty must establish, maintain, and adjust as necessary their boundaries in areas of their work where they choose to work closely with students and devote their extra time and resources to support their students' success. Otherwise, secondary trauma, compassion fatigue, apathy, and burnout are likely to result.[12] For anyone who is engaged in emotional labor it is imperative to establish and maintain boundaries.

Ken talked about his boundaries and a strategy to maintain them. He shared that he is not always perfect at maintaining boundaries and making mental health referrals for students (rather than trying to support his students himself), but he tries to recognize when a professional counselor is a better fit to help a student than he would be. He described his strategy this way:

[M]ost of the time when it comes to mental health-type things, I try not to get too involved in it because, again, that's not my role. But I have physically said [to a student], 'Come with me,' and walked them over and said, "Okay. I don't care who [which counselor] but this is a counseling emergency overriding a [faculty] advising appointment, and I need a counselor."

While Ken did engage in emotional labor, as evidenced by him sharing sentiments like "I care about the student as well. I don't want them to hurt themselves or hurt someone else," he also was cognizant of the importance of boundaries. To that end, he recognized his strengths and his limitations. As someone who struggled with addiction in the past, he noted that one of his strengths is his ability to detect when his students might be struggling, including struggling with mental health issues. He explained:

I also think that because of my experiences [of being in recovery] and because of my background . . . I'm a little bit more aware and hyper vigilant on some of that stuff and I'm able to pick it up a little quicker and say, "Hey. Are you doing okay? Do you need something? Do you need somebody to talk to? You know, what can I do for you?" But all I can do is offer.

Ken taps into his strengths to detect if a student might need help and notes his limitations that "all [he] can do is offer." Offering to direct students to help on campus, rather than trying to directly provide help, is one way Ken maintains his boundaries.

For a variety of reasons, including internal and external reasons, other faculty on campus may not have the capacity to engage in emotional labor and affect-conscious pedagogies like the faculty participants of this study did. Ken explained:

So, it's one of those things where we [faculty] get inundated with so much information anyway about everything else. And most of them [faculty] are going to say, "I'm not a counselor. Not my job." And they're right.

Here, Ken is referencing how a great deal is asked and expected of educators, including community college faculty, that extends beyond typical teaching and learning duties.[13]

Because of the service-oriented nature of teaching, many faculty oblige, but not all do, nor should they. Harriet supported this idea when she stated, "I think that there are a lot of teachers [faculty] who are absolutely not interested at all in getting involved in any of that [nonacademic elements of student life such as mental health]."

Ken also discussed the effect of class frequency and size and faculty disposition on the ability and willingness of faculty to engage in emotional labor. He explained:

> If I was teaching just a regular old class where I'm going to see you for two days a week for 14 weeks, and then I'm never going to see you again, does the average teacher take the time? . . . Go to [a large public institution]. You have 350 students in a lecture class. You don't even know their names. There are professors at this college that treat their classes the same way. Now, there may only be 25 or 30 students in that class. They don't know their names. They don't care what their names are. They're not that invested.

In support of this claim by Ken, Helen mentioned that her institution is "like anyplace [institution of higher education] else. There are some [faculty] that are very black and white, no nonsense, no excuses. That's gonna happen anywhere." By this she meant some faculty are not interested in helping students navigate difficulty, being understanding, or extending students flexibility.

It is also important to mention the structural limitations that some faculty face, whether they are interested in helping students or not. Ken raised the excellent point about the situation of adjunct professors:

> [I] also think about the fact that the majority of our instructors are adjunct. . . . they have full-time jobs elsewhere. They're doing this to pick up some extra money. They don't have time to come to trainings. They don't have time to be invested in all of that.

As this study shows, even though adjunct instructors typically lack the capacity to do more than what is stated in their job descriptions, many *have* gone above and beyond to help their students.

Whether by choice or circumstance, the reality is that not all community college faculty can or will engage in emotional labor in the same way or degree as participants in this study did. Some maintain their own boundaries, while others face structural boundaries that limit their capacity to do more than teach. Another limitation that will be explored in the next section is fear.

## FEAR AND EMOTIONAL LABOR

Lastly, fear can deter faculty from engaging in emotional labor related to students' mental health. Newer faculty, for example, may be surprised by what a student discloses in a paper. If that faculty member feels they ought to do something but do not know what to do, they may become fearful and do nothing as a result. Likewise, they may fear doing the wrong thing. There also may be litigious concerns. Moreover, negative mental health stigmas remain prevalent. The faculty member could become withdrawn from the student and the teaching work as a result. Compassion fatigue and cynicism could also be a deterrent.

Egregiously, some faculty may even make a spectacle of a student's mental health illness or concern. Stephanie explained:

> I think two things might happen with some faculty members [when they encounter a mental health concern]. Number one, I think some don't even want to touch the issue. They'll see it. They'll see evidence in class or they'll see something in an assignment and just say if I ignore it, it'll go away, and they don't even want to touch it. . . . that's fear that if, if I as a professor asks the student about it then they're going to tell me about it and then I'm going to feel like I have to do something. And I don't know what to do. . . . But then I also see many faculty who will approach the student and express concern, uh, and maybe they do know about our wellness counselors, but they maybe don't handle it in the best way [laughs]. Like, uh, for example, . . . a faculty member bringing a student to the front counter and just kind of saying, "She has this and she needs to see someone." [laughs] like right there in the lobby at the counter. Uh, so, yes, it was good intent, but—and knowing, okay, yes, there is this channel if there is this referral but maybe not handling it in the best way. . . . but I still see and I hear people talking, you know, I hear colleagues talking like, "Oh my gosh. Listen to what was in this essay." But not wanting to take it further. Being afraid of it.

Fear and worry circulate around issues like mental health because there is a lot still unknown and misunderstood about it. Without intentional and inclusive professional development about student mental health (which will be discussed in later chapters), it is understandable that faculty and other community college professionals "don't know what to do," as Stephanie shared.

This is a knowledge gap that may be negatively impacting innumerable students, and this is one main reason why studies like the one featured here are essential. To better serve our students, we must make the unknown known, and counter the worry and uncertainty with clarity and confidence about how to serve students best.

## SUMMARY

The faculty in this study engaged in emotional labor, which took many forms. Doing this kind of work was a prerequisite for a faculty member to have cognizance of their students' affect and potential struggles. Using affect-conscious pedagogies precipitated the ability to understand how students were feeling, which certainly can include mental health and mental health concern or illness symptomatology. Emotional labor was carried out in the following ways: knowing students, cultivating relationships with students, coming into solidarity with students, affirming and validating students, listening to students, and being attentive to communicative tones used with students.

There were also examples of how doing emotional labor can yield new insights about honing affect-conscious pedagogies for increased efficacy and continual improvement. The gendered nature of emotional labor—and this study—was considered. The uniqueness of selective, cohort-based programs was also noted in relation to how expectations of emotional labor can be woven into a program's culture. Finally, things that may deter faculty from emotional labor, like fear, compassion fatigue, and cynicism, were mentioned. Engaging in emotional labor laid the foundation for faculty to have perceptions of their students' mental health, which is the focus of the following chapter.

## NOTES

1. Arlie Russell Hochschild, *The Managed Heart: Commercialization of Human Feeling* (Berkeley, CA: University of California Press. 2012; Original work published in 1983).

2. Hochschild, *The Managed Heart.*

3. Julie Beck, "The Concept Creep Of 'Emotional Labor.'" *The Atlantic.* November 26, 2018, https://www.theatlantic.com/family/archive/2018/11/arlie-hochschild -housework-isnt-emotional-labor/576637/.

4. See, for example, Marcia L. Bellas, "Emotional Labor in Academia: The Case of Professors," *The Annals of the American Academy of Political and Social Science* 561 (January 1999): 96–110, https://www.jstor.org/stable/1049284.

5. Brenda G. Kucirka, "Navigating the Faculty-Student Relationship: Interacting with Nursing Students with Mental Health Issues," *Journal of the American Psychiatric Nurses Association* 23, no. 6 (November/December 2017): 393–403, https://doi .org/10.1177/1078390317705451.

6. Kucirka, "Navigating the Faculty-Student Relationship."

7. Kucirka, "Navigating the Faculty-Student Relationship," p. 400.

8. Bellas, "Emotional Labor in Academia."

9. Bellas, "Emotional Labor in Academia."

10. Marion Becker et al., "Students with Mental Illnesses in a University Setting: Faculty and Student Attitudes, Beliefs, Knowledge, and Experiences," *Psychiatric Rehabilitation Journal* 25 no. 4 (Spring 2002): 359–368, https://doi.org/10.1037/

h0095001; Michael T. Kalkbrenner and Kristie L. Carlisle, "Faculty Members and College Counseling: Utility of the REDFLAGS Model. *Journal of College Student Psychotherapy* 35 no. 1 (2021), 70–86, https://doi.org/10.1080/87568225.2019 .1621230; Sarah Ketchen Lipson et al., "Mental Health Conditions Among Community College Students: A National Study of Prevalence and Use of Treatment Services," *Psychiatric Services* 72, no. 10 (October 2021): 1126–1133, https://doi.org /10.1176/appi.ps.202000437.

11. Kelsey Backels and Inese Wheeler, "Faculty Perceptions of Mental Health Issues Among College Students," *Journal of College Student Development* 42 no. 2 (2001): 173.

12. Anna Kariou et al., "Emotional Labor and Burnout Among Teacher: A Systematic Review," *International Journal of Environmental Research and Public Health* 18 no. 23 (December 2021): 12760, https://doi.org/10.3390%2Fijerph182312760.

13. Leslie D. Gonzales and David F. Ayers, "The Convergence of Institutional Logics on the Community College Sector and the Normalization of Emotional Labor: A New Theoretical Approach for Considering the Community College Faculty Labor Expectations," *The Review of Higher Education* 41 no. 3 (Spring 2018): 455–478, https://doi.org/10.1353/rhe.2018.0015.

## Chapter 7

# Rejecting the Monolith

On the prevalence of mental health issues among students: "I think it's huge."

–Eve

"A friend of mine teaches economics, right? College level. Doesn't teach any developmental [courses]. His experience is totally different from mine. . . . We rarely share students. . . . he just sees a completely different population. My experience is much more, with the struggle and strife of, you know, low skills, low socioeconomics, all the stressors associated with poverty, and all that stuff."

–Suzie

In general, the participants in this study noted the high prevalence of mental health concerns among their students. A full participant-by-participant articulation of prevalence is provided within table 4.1. Faculty used terms and phrases like *huge*, *every class*, and *rampant* to describe the prevalence. And these data were collected in 2017, before the global COVID-19 pandemic, which has since negatively exacerbated the community college student mental health landscape.

Joy said, "I mean, every single semester, I'm dealing with students where mental health issues come out in some way that I'm gonna have to intervene." She discussed a recent situation where a student with low vision became very anxious about the pace of a class. Joy was diligent in accommodations but could tell the student was becoming anxious during the class session. She mentioned that within every class, there are instances of students whose mental health concerns are so great their academic abilities are negatively affected. Joy shared that she had one student who "had to do a group project, and she just did not show up to do the presentation because she couldn't handle [the] anxiety."

Community college students who have or may have a mental health issue are not all the same. Monolithic views of this sort were rejected by the faculty within this study. Alternatively, a perceptual typology or model (here used synonymously) that showcased the spectrum of students dealing with mental health issues was built from the study's early interviews and member-checked during subsequent interviewees.

Member checking involves asking the participants of a study to *check* the accuracy of the data they created, and it can sometimes extend to asking participants to *check* the researcher's interpretations of those data, or the results of the study. Though contested, member checking is one way some qualitative researchers promote trustworthiness within their studies.[1] It can add to a study's validity. This opens opportunities for participants to further articulate meanings and contribute to researchers' understandings of the topic under study.

Based on faculty perceptions and verified by faculty participants, there are five types of students with mental health issues. These types are fluid and nonrigid, however, and students can flow easily among them. They are as follows and defined below: (1) disclosed issue or diagnosis, (2) undisclosed (possible) issue or diagnosis, (3) situational struggle, (4) mediation through medication, and (5) distressing behavior.

1. Disclosed Issue or Diagnosis. These are students who have an issue or diagnosis and disclose that issue or diagnosis. Disclosure came, for example, in the form of an in-class announcement, a class paper, an email, a formal letter from the disability office and a follow-up conversation about the letter, or a one-on-one meeting.
2. Undisclosed (possible) Issue or Diagnosis. These are students who may or may not have a diagnosis and do not disclose. These students present red flags,[2] or symptoms, related to mental illness.
3. Situational Struggle. These are students who, because of a difficult and stressful life event or circumstance, experience a situational mental health issue such as anxiety and/or depression. They did not have a diagnosis, and they may or may not disclose what they are experiencing. Yet, red flags, or symptoms, are being presented. This is a time-bound experience.
4. Mediation through Medication. These are students who, in anticipation of a stressful academic experience such as a test or in-class presentation, seek medication from a general practitioner or family doctor to cope with the stress of the situation. These students may or may not have a diagnosis, and they may or may not disclose these actions or how they

are feeling. Many faculty associated these actions with a lack of coping skills.

5. Distressing Behavior. These are students who may or may not have a diagnosis and may or may not disclose, but because of severe behavioral problems that may or may not be related to mental health, they are unable to continue functioning in the community college environment.

Faculty discussed that each one of the student types above requires a certain set of approaches in terms of support, referral, and help giving.

On the one hand, it is important to realize typologies are mental models that help classify information into categories meant to convey and assist with understanding. Such models make it easier to manage and digest a lot of complicated information. On the other hand, presenting complicated information in the form of a typology can be essentializing. It may dismiss or render invisible important details, contexts, situations, temporality, and other critical factors. Readers are encouraged to remember and appreciate that students are all people who live complicated lives *and* to use this typology to enhance their understanding and make sense of student experiences.

Additionally, this typology was built from interactions with community college faculty members. Were it built from interactions with student affairs professionals, members of the president's or chancellor's cabinet, or students themselves, the model might look different. If it were built from a different group of community college faculty, the typology might also look differently—or not exist at all.

However, the typology fully presented in this chapter can be useful in understanding faculty perceptions of and experiences with community college students' mental health. Readers are encouraged to intentionally use the model in praxis with care and thoughtful consideration. Local context is critical. Further research is also necessary to evaluate the efficacy of the model. The literature on community college student mental health is sparse yet growing, and other researchers are encouraged to take up these ongoing inquiries.

## DISCLOSED ISSUE OR DIAGNOSIS

As mentioned above, there are many ways students may disclose having a mental health concern or issue or diagnosed mental health disorder or illness. This may include volunteering the information during class, sharing it in an email or other electronic message, providing an accommodation letter from disability services, discussing it in an in-person meeting, video conference, or phone call, and writing about it in a course paper, discussion forum, or other type of written assignment.

Carolyn mentioned being intentional about making space for students to disclose (personal) information that would help her understand and work with them. For example, she asked students to complete index cards with this sort of information (by student choice) and regularly held one-on-one faculty-student conferences.

About disclosure, Rebecca shared she has had students who have announced on day one of her developmental English class "I'm gonna sit in the front because I have ADHD, and I need to pay attention." Some students are unbothered by disclosure and readily do so. But others may not be so inclined. I should note here that while ADHD is considered a mental illness by some entities such as the National Alliance on Mental Illness (NAMI), ADHD is also a form of neurodiversity and can also be considered a disability for which students can seek accommodations.

Pam noted that "there's a handful in the class that have . . . serious, chronic mental health issues. . . . Be it anxiety, OCD [obsessive compulsive disorder], depression." She shared that when a student discloses a particular issue, she believes that it is a sign they feel safe within the classroom. Pam further explained, "Sometimes students will just come out in class and say 'I have this. I've been diagnosed with this.' . . . I think it decreases the stigma. I really do."

When talking about the typology, Joy discussed how she really emphasizes resources available to students, disability disclosures, documentation, and accommodations, and the importance of self-advocacy. She takes a relational and empathic approach to the conversation at the start of classes in hopes that students will feel compelled to share if necessary:

> I have a very frank, open, honest discussion with my students . . . If you've given me a letter, please come and talk to me 'cause I wanna make sure I'm doing everything I can for you. . . . So I try to start that relationship off. Like, please come and talk to me. I can be supportive if I know what's going on and you come and talk to me . . . I want everyone to be successful.

Disclosure through email was mentioned by Geraldine, who also emphasizes the importance of communication, building rapport, and making use of available resources. She explained she has students whose typical past "interactions with educational professionals have not been positive," so she really tries to build a "positive rapport" with students by learning their names, learning something about each student, and engaging in "a little chit-chat before class."

She has found that taking steps to get to know her students in these ways, leaning into emotional labor with them, and using affect-conscious pedagogical techniques all help students feel comfortable sharing with her any mental health issues with which they might be struggling. It may take a little time, and they may be hesitant to share face-to-face, but eventually they email her because, as she explained, "I always say 'Look, if you don't communicate with me, then I don't know what's going on.'" She tells her students and shows her students that she cares, and in turn, they trust her and confide in her.

Some courses and course assignments may facilitate a student disclosure as well. An example may be classes where students are asked to write about their lives. Stephanie explained how students will often share within journal entries:

> In our first-year seminar classes, we have what we call journals. It's asking students to take the content and apply it to their lives and reflect. And in every class, I have several students who use life examples of mental illness. "And I have this, I have this, I was diagnosed with this, I've struggled with this." . . . And so I know they've been through the system. They've had some sort of diagnosis. They maybe had treatment. They've had meds or whatever. They—you can tell from the language that they know what they're talking about.

This experience resonated with Suzie, who teaches developmental English. She mentioned that one of the first assignments in her course is a personal narrative essay, and students "frequently reveal" mental health issues in that assignment. She described what students have shared as "unbelievable." Students have a lot to share. She explained; "It's almost like there's no filter." Though not intentionally designed to gauge student mental health issues, that first assignment allows her to "pick up on a lot of that" and keeps her abreast of and attuned to student issues.

Pam discussed how students often disclose during individual meetings. Often, conversations about coursework can lead to discussion about factors affecting the student's academic performance: "They might come in to meet with you and just kind of break down crying in your office. . . . that usually leads to a disclosure of 'It's not just school.' . . . 'I have this diagnosis.'" Camille discussed a similar scenario:

> I try to talk to them. Basically, not in front of anybody, but I ask, "How you doing? How are things going? Are you understanding the assignment?" . . . Or, "I noticed that you haven't been coming to class." Or "I notice you're coming in late, is everything okay?" And they usually will, 99 percent of the time, they'll talk to me. They'll just start talking. You know? And I say, "Well, come to my office, and we can close the door a little bit." And sometimes they start crying.

By opening the conversation in a care-centered and nonthreatening way, Camille creates a space within which students may feel comfortable sharing what they are experiencing. And sometimes that experience includes navigating a mental health issue or concern.

## UNDISCLOSED (POSSIBLE) ISSUE OR DIAGNOSIS

According to participants in this study, the most prevalent student group is the group of students who do not disclose their mental health issues. Sandie believes most students with mental health concerns are "undiagnosed" and "unaware" they have issues themselves, which naturally means they lack official support from any disability services on campus. Harriet agreed; she noted:

> I see the largest category of students of who I think [*sic*] are highly anxious and are depressed. I don't think they're doing anything about it. Anxiety, definitely, and I understand some that's perfectly normal in the classroom. But, I have the feeling it, sort of, almost paralyzes them, in some cases.

Ken said many of his students do not think their problems are serious enough to disclose or students feel shameful about what they are experiencing.

Suzie described how she would approach a student who was struggling within her course or showing some signs of mental health concerns as follows, noting negative mental health stigmas as a barrier to disclosure:

> I don't ask, you know, "Do you have mental illness?" But I, but I say, you know, "How are you? What's going on?" "Do you think there's a reason why—why do you think you're not, you know, doing this?" And a lot of students will volunteer it. A lot of students, especially, I think, once they feel that you're asking for the right reasons, they will volunteer it. Um, but, you know, a lot of students are very worried about the stigma.

Joy explained her approach in a similar way to Suzie, gently sharing her concern, offering support, and then providing accountability, if necessary:

> What I would do is I would try to pull them [student] and say, "You know, I have some concerns." Um, if I'm seeing their academic work, I might bring that up. "You know, I see your performance in class, but then I get your academic work. It's kind of late. Um, I really want you to be successful here. I'm wondering if there's something you need help with or some way I can support you." . . . And sometimes that will break the ice, and then I'll be able to help them with that. And usually it does [break the ice]. It's pretty rare that I get a student who just can't be worked with. Um, I've had one or two of those where I've had to say, "Look, you know, I've had a couple talks. I've tried." Then I say, "I have to make sure you understand that these are the requirements of the class, and if

you need help or support, I, I'm willing to help you with that, but the other half of this is you've got to do the work."

If a student misses two classes in a row, Stephanie will email, call, and place an alert in the software system used to communicate with the student's advisor and other faculty. She does the same thing if a student's assignment is more than one week late. If a student is present in class, she will talk with them at the start of class.

Another barrier to student disclosure is worry that they will receive differential treatment or will not be recommended or hired because of a mental illness or concern. Ken, who teaches respiratory therapy, said:

> My students aren't going to come in and say, "Oh well, you know, I'm dysthymic with, you know, periods of schizophrenic outrage." I'm going to have trepidation about them in clinical, and how are you going to be in clinical, and am I going to treat them differently? I would hope not, but I might. And somebody who isn't as aware as me is definitely going to treat them differently.

This barrier to disclosure is important for faculty, especially those whose programs or courses lead directly to work. Faculty must consider the professional, ethical, and even legal obligations they or their students may have with regards to mental health screening, diagnosis, and treatment. Faculty in these kinds of programs ought to work collaboratively to build clear policies and procedures regarding this issue. Through orientation, coursework, and advising, students should be made aware of these important considerations related to their futures.

## SITUATIONAL STRUGGLE

Tess noted that many students frequently experience situation-based and time-bound difficulties that affect their mental health and cause them to struggle. Examples may include having a car accident, experiencing a house fire, mourning the death of a loved one, or navigating a relationship issue or divorce.

Tess received an email from a student who told her, "I can't make it to class tomorrow . . . My transmission blew up." What resulted for this student was more than merely transportation difficulties. Tess explained the student experienced a lot of anxiety and insomnia while wrestling with the concern and uncertainty about whether they could find a way to repair their car. As Camille succinctly summarized, students are "just trying to make ends meet. That puts so much pressure [on them]."

Like Tess, Rose also noted that many students experience situational struggles. She shared an example of how a traumatic situation can lead to attrition for students. Rose had one student who had taken a course with her, "attended class regularly," and did very well. The student enjoyed the course so much that she shared with Rose that she was excited about taking a second class with her.

Rose shared that the student "showed up the first class and then disappeared." She went on to tell the story of what transpired. The student and her daughter had been living with a man who attempted suicide in front of them. This was a serious and traumatic event, which resulted in the student not returning to the course. Rose explained that "it took her [student] six weeks before she could come tell me about that, you know? To withdraw from the class . . . that, that was why." Traumatic events happen—some absolutely devastating, like the one Rose described—and they most definitely impact student mental health and persistence.

Sandie expressed a deep concern for students experiencing situational mental health issues, noting that, if not addressed, the situation could continue or worsen, which means the mental health issues could become long-term. This phenomenon is an example of how the student groups within the typology are porous and nonrigid. If not resolved over time, situational struggles can become longstanding. Sandie shared that she had a student who was experiencing bedbugs, which led to, in her view, "situational depression" and crisis. She then explained:

> I think the problem for me is that I see somebody in that situation, and I know that without help or aid, that that crisis is going to continue, which is going to create a long-term clinical depression, which is gonna worsen. And this person doesn't have access to quality mental health [care].

This situation highlights how a relatively simple problem with a simple solution (like having bedbugs) can become a crisis because of systemic issues, such as poverty and poor health care options. Too often these problems do not get resolved, and student mental health and success suffer as a result.

Students within this category (i.e., situational struggles) can experience mental health concerns with a broad range of severity. Some students may experience mild depression for a week after a breakup, for example, while others may experience crisis while on campus. Ken gave an example of the latter. He had a student he knew well whose sister was dying of cancer and who was also taking care of her sister's kids.

The student confided in Ken and expressed anxiety, asking him "How am I going to do this?" and stating "I don't know what I'm going to do." He helped her take a breath after meeting with her and shared with her,

Okay. You're—you do zero self-care. You've already been depressed. I know that you're already medicated. . . . Basically, you're having a meltdown. And no, I don't feel that you should leave here and go get in a car and drive home. Let me take you over to talk to somebody.

He helped calm her down and connect her with the support she needed at that moment.

To summarize, situational struggles are a part of life. They are to be expected. But for many community college students, especially those who may be struggling with financial insecurity and poverty, these situational struggles may be a regular occurrence.

## MEDIATION THROUGH MEDICATION

Psychotropic medications such as antidepressants, stimulants, antipsychotics, and mood stabilizers are an important part of mental health treatment. While negative stigmas about this type of treatment exist, many college students are prescribed and regularly take these medications. Without specific prompting, many faculty discussed student use of psychotropic medication.

Some faculty believe some students were using medication to manage the normal stressors of college life because they lacked the necessary knowledge and skills to cope with these stressors without them. Some of these stressors may include heavy reading assignments, lengthy tests based on memorizing large quantities of information, and performing under pressure in clinical settings.

To be clear, faculty differentiated between students who were regularly taking psychotropic medications prescribed by a mental health or health care provider to manage one or more diagnosed mental health disorder or illness and students who accessed prescriptions for psychotropic medications through a family doctor or general practitioner because of a self-determined need. For example, a student may request a prescription for an antianxiety medication meant to address acute anxiety, which would then be taken prior to class in anticipation of experiencing high levels of anxiety in the space.

Related to this circumstance, Tess, who teaches business courses, shared, "I would say there's a population of students who just lack coping skills" and don't know how to "manage stressful situations." She shared that she's heard students say, "I have a job interview, so I've got to take medication for that." According to Tess, this is most prevalent among her younger students. Camille agreed and noted seeing a relationship between perfectionism and using medication:

I'm looking at these classes, and I see some of the younger [students] that had to go on medication. I think the ones that expect the absolute best out of themselves, they have such high standards for themselves, tend to have the issues, too. The ones that have seen that they're not perfect, and have dealt with that already, tend to be able to deal with the stresses a little bit better.

Helen noted that, in her experience, the incidence of students seeking medication to cope with stressful situations, including academic and other events and circumstances, has risen over time, which she has noticed in her role within disabilities services as well.

There is nothing wrong with taking medication to manage mental health issues. In fact, for some it is lifesaving. That this student group contains more younger students than older students may be related to the fact that many mental issues, illnesses, and disorders first present during early adulthood. However, some participants took the position that if coping skills were enhanced, the need for medication predicated by stressful circumstances (including events faculty saw as routine in many cases) would dissipate.

However, coping skills are often learned in therapy. Therapy can be expensive, and it can come with severe negative stigmas within certain cultures. Therefore, accessing and using psychotropic medication in this way could be framed as a rational choice for many students. While not brought up within the interviews, students' use of medication to manage mental health through nonstructured or illegal means is also a part of this story. Self-medicating with nonprescribed medications or illicit substances was not a part of the conversations with participants. Yet, it is likely happening among community college students and should be further researched.[3]

## Academic Program

On the topic of student mental health and student use of medication, it is important to consider the role of the academic program. Pam teaches within the nursing program, a selective, cohort-based program that is known for challenging course content and clinical experiences that may be traumatic. Many of her students shared with her that they went on antidepressants after their first semester in the nursing program because of the stress.

Pam explained that college can be full of triggers for students—some courses and programs more than others. For example, she shared, "One of the lectures that I teach is about suicide. And I would say, at least every semester, one time, at least one student is touched by suicide. And . . . during that lecture, I see them in the back, crying."

Christina, who works within the sonography program, another selective, cohort-based program, said she's heard students mention that over half to three-quarters of a class were "on some type of medication" because they were "under so much stress." She was dumbfounded by the number of students going that route. She shared, "I think it is huge that these students had to see a physician to get medication to help control their stress levels."

Research set within the four-year sector and focused on selective and intense programs such as nursing can help shed light on student mental health. For example, transitioning to college coupled with the stress of a nursing program may place students at increased risk for depression.[4] Going into and becoming immersed in clinical settings is often difficult for students,[5] with some students reporting trouble relaxing and difficulty sleeping.[6]

Academic programs matter to student mental health. Kucirka said "[n]ursing education occurs in a rigorous, high stakes learning environment. Therefore, it is not surprising that nursing students have been found to have increased anxiety and depression in comparison to the 'general' college student population."[7] Data from student mental health screenings and help-seeking behavior surveys should also be differentiated by academic program, as program-specific interventions may be most effective in providing students with the resources they need.

What concerned Harriet, who teaches English, was the potential lack of professional oversight of students taking medication in what might be thought of as a casualized way. It should be noted that implicit in these comments is the notion that long-term usage of these medications is negative or harmful and that clear lines should be drawn between grief and depression. She remarked:

> When I was talking earlier about students being on medication, I think my concern there is that there isn't monitoring. And, so they continue—they continue with that medication without, I think, any expectation of moving beyond it. And, lots of times I'm not sure that the medication is right for them. They're not feeling well, but that's what the doctors prescribed. It's, sort of, like this, this quick, band-aid, or that they go [seek medication] for what is a normal event.

Taking medication rather than using other methods to manage stress and/or mental health concerns or illness was seen as an easier route to take by Camille, who said the "medication is so easy to get that instead of working different ways to deal with stress they go right towards that [medication]."

But it may not be so easy for all students. Suzie, who teaches developmental English, had a contrasting viewpoint regarding this category. She wondered who the types of students would be "who would go to the doctor and say, 'I need, I'd like some medication to help with this.'" She shared, "A lot of my students get their medical care from the ER, you know? [They] don't have doctors, don't have insurance." Though she was "sure it happens some," opting to seek medication to counter stress seemed to Suzie as more of a "privileged response" for a select group of students. Rebecca, who also teaches developmental English, concurred with Suzie's explanation.

Those who teach courses with no prerequisites such as developmental courses (like Suzie and Rebecca) may have a better sense of what it means to be an open-access institution. Those students who are admitted into selective programs may be able to do so, in part, because of some level of privilege related to their background and socioeconomic status. Students may possess the social and cultural capital necessary to access psychotropic medications because of that privilege.

For example, a student may go to a family doctor who is a friend of the family or neighbor (social capital), which may compel that doctor to comply with the student's request without encouraging other or complementary approaches like therapy. The student may be conversant about different types, names, and manufacturers of the medications by having the ability to look up such information online using a laptop or tablet (cultural capital). Based on Suzie's excerpt above, students within her developmental English courses may not possess those forms of capital.

Stephanie, who teaches first-year seminar courses, which have no prerequisites, provided additional evidence that there may be a relationship between this category of students and academic program. She said:

> I don't know that I have personally been aware of a student in the . . . situation where you know, something related to school caused them to seek [medical] help rather than, you know, lack of coping skills. I definitely see students who don't have the coping skills, but I think what I've mostly seen is that they actually fail. Like whatever happens it happens. They have a failure and then maybe they do go seek help. I don't know that I personally have been aware of anyone who, uh, says, "Well, school is really tough and I'm going to go to my family doctor and ask for like Ativan or something." I haven't necessarily seen that.

This example, again, seems to contrast with what was shared by those teaching in highly selective, cohort-based programs.

## DISTRESSING BEHAVIOR

About halfway through the interviews, when speaking with Joy, who is a licensed clinical psychologist, this fifth category was created, which she articulated in the following way:

> There's another group of students. They're the people with the serious mental health problems. There's not a lot of them, thank God. Um, who are not very

functional, who come onto the campus, who disrupt our class, who make other people afraid of them. And then become a challenge because every semester, we're discussing them at a behavioral meeting as to what should be the next step. . . . Um, but more problematic is at what point do we say, "You can't be here," You know, and these are people who, eventually, we come to find out because often they don't disclose right away that they have chronic schizophrenia . . . paranoid schizophrenia . . . bipolar disorder with psychotic features. . . . and you've got five students go to the dean because "I can't be in class with this person. They're scaring the hell out of me."

Joy went on to say there are very few students who fit into this category.

In fact, many faculty participants had no experience with this type of student whose distressing behavior may make it untenable and impossible for them to persist at the college. Furthermore, it can be very difficult and take a lot of time to come to the point of dismissing a student from the institution.

In addition to teaching courses, Sandie also worked as a tutor. She told a story about a particular student's behavior that was distressing and "scary." The pseudonym name "Jacob" will be used to protect the student and faculty member's identity. Jacob often frequented the tutoring lab where she worked. One day he came by and asked if any of the tutors there wanted to go to lunch. In her retelling of what happened, she shared that she told the student, "You know what, [Jacob], we're working, and so we can't go to lunch with you. You can go to lunch and come back if you need help with a paper, but this is our job."

According to Sandie, Jacob reacted in very scary and disturbing ways. She explained, "He completely became unhinged and verbally abusive." He screamed, yelled, and used a variety of expletives, including "Fuck you. You're not my fucking friends," before he stormed out. Sandie immediately went to her supervisor and told her what happened.

Because Jacob was a student who visited the tutoring lab often, Sandie, her colleagues, and her supervisor knew him and knew a little about his background. They knew that he was a student veteran and was possibly managing post-traumatic stress issues. The tutoring lab "filled out the appropriate report" to share what happened and the college's Office of Veterans' Affairs reached out to Jacob to address the problematic behavior he displayed at the tutoring lab and provide him with more support, including increasing the frequency of his counseling sessions.

Sandie explained what happened after that and the impact of that distressing day:

We didn't see him again. I don't know if he was embarrassed. I don't know. I don't know what happened, but it was scary. It was scary in one of those ways where I think "Gosh, the reason he so messed up is because of what he did for us [as a veteran]." You know, and I don't know. It was really kind of hard.

Whether the student persisted or not was unknown to Sandie, but his distressing behavior meant an intervention was necessary. As is evident in Sandie's commentary, taking actions that seem disciplinary is not easy. None of the participants in this study wanted to see a student fail or be unable to persist. However, the safety of students (including the student exhibiting distressing behavior), personnel, and the overall campus community is paramount.

Justin shared an evocative story that warrants consideration involving a student he had never met before who burst into his classroom one day. A full description of what happened follows below to provide a sense of what it might have been like to have been in his shoes. He said this was the scariest situation he has encountered as a faculty member. First, to provide context, he shared a little about a different student in his class who played a role in the story. He shared:

Soon after the first Gulf War, I had a woman in my class, African American woman, who, who was there, who [fought in that war] . . . And she always came in, sat right in front, she was very prim, very proper, always very, you know, just a very excellent person, excellent student, you know, just on top of everything, had all her assignments done exactly on time, exactly the way I asked her to, I mean, she was that kind of person.

Then he shared what happened the day of the incident:

I'll never forget, it was six weeks into the semester, and I was lecturing. And I'm standing at the podium, and all of a sudden this very, very large woman, this was, you know, 7:00 at night, bursts into the room and came walking right at me. I had never seen this woman before in my life. And she got about maybe, I don't know, eight feet away from me, stopped, and said, "I'm taking this class." And it was [six weeks into the term, so] too late to take the class, right? So, um, and then she just plopped herself down [in a seat].

Justin wasn't sure what to do. He told his class that it was time to take a break. He continued:

I had 25 students in this class. [I told them], "I think we need to take a break, take a fifteen-minute break." The student that was in the front here, the woman in the army, she just sat there. I said, "You're not going to take a break?" She goes, "I got your back," just like that [laughs].

It was both concerning and reassuring to Justin that the army veteran in his class also sensed danger and was there to help him out as needed.

Justin proceeded cautiously. He asked the student who burst into his class-room to step into the hallway to have a conversation. She responded in an abrupt and brusque tone, "All right, I'll talk to you in the hallway, [but] I'm gonna be taking this class," which further unnerved him.

In the classroom where he was teaching, there was a button available to faculty to push if they ever needed technology help. Discreetly, he told the student veteran in his class, "Do me a favor, hit the help button." He explained:

> Now, the help button goes to the IT people [laughs]. I, I don't have any button for security, I got nothing, right? So, all I got is me, some lady that's in the army, and a 400-pound woman ready to kill me.

When he walked out into the hallway with the student, he was even more unnerved. He explained he saw "this little man and two little kids, and they were standing against the wall. And they had their hands down, their faces down, and I'm like, "What is going on here?" He told the student, "Ma'am, I really can't allow you to be in here until you bring me something from the Bursar or the Registrar Office that says you're signed up for this class and you're paid up."

The student told him, "My kids and my husband are gonna see that I, that they can be proud of me, that I take these classes and I can pass this stuff." Justin explained:

> It was her family standing in the hallway. And, uh, I said, "Ma'am, I'm sure they're proud of you already, and I'm sure you could pass this class, I have no question about that. I just can't let you in here, and if you keep insisting that you're gonna be in here." And then here's when the IT guy shows up [laughs].

At that point, the IT person called security, and the situation was eventually diffused. But here again is an example of aberrant behavior from a student who may have been managing mental health issues that a faculty member and other students not only observed, but also experienced and that left an impact on them.

A note about violence should be made here. While there have been some horrific acts of violence committed by students on community college cam-puses, violence is endemic to society. Plenty of acts of violence are commit-ted every day for reasons having nothing to do with mental health. At the same time, campus safety is vital; it is necessary for learning. This type does warrant serious attention. But at the same time, this type includes a very small population of students. Again, community college students who are managing mental health issues are not a monolithic group. This typology is one step in helping practitioners and others see the many nuances surrounding student mental health issues.

## SUMMARY

According to the faculty participants within this study and the extant literature, prevalence of mental health concerns and illnesses is high. Community college students managing these issues are not a monolithic group, however, and this cannot be overemphasized.

Within this chapter, a five-part typology was articulated, built directly from the interviews conducted. The categories within the typology are not absolute. Instead, they are fluid and porous, which should be considered when using the model in praxis. Faculty expressed specific ways of working with, supporting, and acting as referral agents dependent on type.

While this typology provides a helpful mental model, students should not be essentialized into types. Students are complex, with life histories, vast experience, and tapestries of identities. As each student is unique, so is each situation. This model should be applied using contextual competency and care.[8] While the efficacy of this model may be bound to those who played a part in creating it, it is likely transferrable to other contexts. Others are encouraged to apply, interrogate, and adjust the model through practice and inquiry. The next chapter is focused on how these faculty navigated institutional structures and systems related to community college student mental health.

## NOTES

1. Linda Birt et al., "Member Checking: A Tool to Enhance Trustworthiness or Merely a Nod to Validation?" *Qualitative Health Research* 26 no. 13 (November 2016): 1802–1811, https://doi.org/10.1177/1049732316654870.

2. See Michael T. Kalkbrenner, "Recognizing and Supporting Students with Mental Health Disorders: The REDFLAGS Model," *Journal of Education and Training* 3 no. 1 (February 2016), http://dx.doi.org/10.5296/jet.v3i1.8141.

3. Dorothy Wallis et al., "Predicting Self-Medication with Cannabis in Young Adults with Hazardous Cannabis Use," *International Journal of Environmental Research and Public Health* 19 no. 3 (February 2022): 1850, https://doi.org/10.3390/ijerph19031850.

4. Wanda M. Chernomas and Carla Shapiro, "Stress, Depression, and Anxiety Among Undergraduate Nursing Students," *International Journal of Nursing Education Scholarship* 10 no. 1 (2013): 255–266, https://doi.org/10.1515/ijnes-2012-0032.

5. Cristobal Jimenez et al., "Stress and Health in Novice and Experienced Nursing Students," *Journal of Advanced Nursing* 66 no. 2 (February 2010): 442–455, https://doi.org/10.1111/j.136-2648.2009.05183.x.

6. Laura C. Dzurec et al., "First-Year Nursing Students' Accounts of Reasons for Student Depression," *Journal of Nursing Education* 46 no. 12 (December 2007): 545–551, https://doi.org/10.3928/01484834-20071201-04.

7. Brenda G. Kucirka, "Navigating the Faculty-Student Relationship: Interacting with Nursing Students with Mental Health Issues," *Journal of the American Psychiatric Nurses Association* 23, no. 6 (November/December 2017): 394, https://doi.org/10.1177/1078390317705451.

8. Pamela L. Eddy, "A Holistic Perspective of Leadership Competencies," *New Directions for Community Colleges* 2012 no. 159 (Autumn/Fall 2012): 29–39, https://doi.org/10.1002/cc.20024.

# Chapter 8

# Navigating Institutional Structures and Systems

"I do everything I can to help [students] succeed . . . I won't break any rules, but I'll bend them if I have to, to help them succeed."

–Martin

A variety of scholars have examined how students must navigate burdensome and complicated institutional structures and systems throughout their education experience.[1] From the way colleges are organizationally and academically structured, to how siloed or aligned campus functions and services might be, to how confusing or inconsistent institutional policies and practices are and more, the structures and systems at a college greatly influence students and the student experience.[2]

This is no different for faculty members and their experiences. However, it is important to note that much less research has been conducted on the challenges faculty have faced while attempting to navigate their colleges' systems and structures. This chapter is meant to address that gap by showcasing the perspectives of faculty who have attempted to navigate their college's systems and structures in an effort to support students with mental health concerns.

One of the most prominent frustrations voiced by faculty interviewed for this study was the lack of follow-up or feedback from their college after they referred a student to counseling and/or to the college's Behavioral Intervention Team (BIT). BITs are comprised of a dedicated group of campus personnel who receive, assess, and sometimes act upon information about students exhibiting worrisome behavior. These teams are concerned with maintaining a safe campus environment and supporting students whose behaviors warrant swift attention or intervention. Many campuses have an online portal where personnel can make a report to the BIT.

Silence from the college postreferral prevented faculty from feeling aware, connected, or a sense of closure regarding their actions on behalf of a student. Helen said "I think once it [referral] gets into that system [counseling and/or BIT] and that system feels the situation is resolved, then it's done." Helen's use of the word *think* shows a sense of being unsure, and her reference to *the system* conjures images of a bureaucratic machine devoid of humanness.

Pam made a similar comment regarding referrals to counselors at the college. She said, "Once they're [students are] referred to counseling—we don't get to—we're not in on it." Faculty like Helen and Pam who made referrals expressed frustration about this process and the lack of connection and closure seemingly endemic to it. They care about their students and want to know if their students are going to be alright. The lack of follow-up was a source of frustration and angst.

Furthermore, many faculty viewed the BIT as a punitive body. Some faculty noted they would rather manage student issues and concerns on their own, without any sort of intervention from the BIT. Faculty worried that having a referral on a student's permanent record would be damaging to students later. The BIT was seen as a last resort that could be ultimately harmful to the student. Instead of feeling connected and a part of a team at the college, some faculty felt very much on their own and, worse, distrustful of staff and structures (like the BIT) at the college that were supposed to support students.

## REFERRAL TO COUNSELING

Some faculty were frustrated when they encouraged a student to go to counseling for support, but then not knowing—and not being able to find out—whether the student accessed the service. For example, Sandie shared a story of when she had a student in her office, and in conversation he mentioned he only feels comfortable "when he was holding a gun." She was alarmed by his comment but tried to show care and empathy.

In her interview, Sandie relayed that she told him it was "a little concerning" to hear him say he only feels comfortable if he is holding a gun and asked him, "Would you be willing to maybe talk about that a little bit more?" According to Sandie, his response was an abrupt "No!" She responded calmly that she understood, and he should know that, if he changes his mind and would like to talk to someone, there are services on campus for students. She explained:

> I gave him a brochure for counseling and advising. And I was also clear with him, you can always come and see me, and I'd be happy to go with him there

if he'd feel more comfortable. Um, I don't know if he ever followed up on the brochure or not.

Jody told a story about a student who had been struggling in one of her courses. She found out later that the student had attempted suicide. After talking with the student at length about her concern and the availability of counseling on campus, Jody asked her "[a]re you willing to go down and get an appointment?," and the student finally agreed. They walked across campus to make the appointment together, which was the last week of classes for that term.

Jody mentioned she "kind of felt in a way that I'm not sure she was going to go [to the appointment]. I was hoping that everything was going to turn out okay." After a few days, Jody "did go back to the counseling office to ask them if she did follow-up with her appointment, and they couldn't tell me." This was a point of frustration, as Jody was growing more and more concerned about the student.

A few days after checking in with counseling personnel, Jody learned the student had attempted suicide and was involuntarily committed to a mental health institution. The student was hospitalized for about a month. Jody explained that the student was "holding an F in her class" but she decided to " put an incomplete on file." Jody was willing to "work with her if she would like to come back and try to finish out her work," noting "I won't fail her."

Jody mentioned the student "did come back after a month" and "she did complete, and she passed." Jody went on to explain that she was unsure whether there was a missed opportunity to help the student or even prevent a suicide attempt because of the lack of communication between campus personnel. Jody said she "shared with [the counseling staff] what did happen, and I know that in reverse they can't share anything back." She concluded by saying "I think this girl did tell me she was supposed to follow-up with her . . . psychologist. I don't know if she did or not. So, I was very sad about that when I heard that that [suicide attempt] happened."

Phoebe provided another example. Because of Phoebe's former career as a lawyer, she is very aware of off-campus resources to which she often refers students. For students who may otherwise be referred to counseling, Phoebe often refers them directly to the community agency or advocate the student may need.

Faculty have varied knowledge about what is available in the community, varied types of relationships (or nonrelationships) with helpful community agencies and/or individuals, and varied skill sets regarding referral. For example, an adjunct human services faculty member may feel more comfortable with referring to off-campus resources than on-campus ones.

In some cases, this may help students avoid an extra step in the help-seeking process by accessing the appropriate agency or individual from the start. Phoebe said "issues that I've dealt with are often battered women. And I refer them directly to the domestic abuse legal services. I've refer[red] people to lawyers all the time." She went on to say "it's been a while since I referred anybody to counseling."

As is evident through the above accounts, faculty expressed some concern and frustration about navigating the referral to counseling process. There were frustrations about lacking feedback and follow-up once a referral had been made. Legal and professional obligations about confidentiality regarding counseling and help-seeking notwithstanding, faculty often felt blocked out of the process, leaving them to feel helpless.

Others saw referral to counseling as ineffectual or temporary and instead referred directly to community resources. Yet in the context of supporting students' mental health, referral to counseling was not the only institutional structure or system faculty had to navigate.

## BEHAVIORAL INTERVENTION TEAM REPORTING

The BIT reporting process was another topic brought up by several faculty. Some faculty *and students* viewed BIT reports as penalizing students. Once the report is made, the faculty are effectively *done* with the BIT process. And like the faculty sentiments above, this is seen as problematic, because no direction or guidance is given regarding what happened, how the student is doing, or how to work with the student going forward. Sandie said "[s]o my perception is, it's supportive [the Behavioral Intervention Team], but . . . I feel confident the student perspective—I've had students in class, talking about being *reported* to BIT."

Geraldine noted that if a student's behavior is negatively affecting the safety of the class, she is compelled to make a report. She mentioned always talking with the student first, however. Her understanding of the process was different from and more intricate than other faculty. She explained:

> We can make what's called the BIT report . . . and it either goes to counseling or it goes to discipline, and you can kind of indicate. So, like if, if a student expresses something that I think is a concern, like suicidal or something I might do a BIT report, but I wouldn't say "This is discipline," I will say "This is referral." So, a BIT report can go either way. And it even could just be "I'm documenting this behavior; we don't really need any intervention right now."

Geraldine was an outlier with regards to this thorough and nuanced understanding of the BIT reporting workflow. However, even the documentation of behavior affordance of the BIT reporting process was seen as problematic by some faculty, as will be outlined later in this chapter.

Jody expressed hesitation with making a report to the BIT but did not say a lot about why. She then later went on to explain: "that [hesitation] may be me just because I'd like to try to help them [students] first." To Jody, making a BIT report was akin to no longer being able to help the student. The BIT was viewed as a last resort. She framed making a BIT report as a failure of communication and non-use of problem-solving strategies.

Jody said "I feel that we [people in general] . . . sometimes . . . cause conflict, and we shouldn't be causing conflict because [of] our inability to have constructive conversation." Again, here she is alluding to making a BIT report because of an inability to deal with a given situation through effective communication. She summed up her sentiments by sharing, "I feel like that I am putting them [students reported to the BIT] into a disadvantage." Here again, this passage suggests making a BIT report is seen as punitive for students.

Suzie expressed strong feelings about the BIT process; she noted a sense of betrayal and a resultant feeling of being quite upset:

> The notion that I can fill out a behavioral intervention, um, form, online, but I cannot know what steps have been taken with that student [is a problem]. I am not informed, and the student keeps coming back to my class, and I'm being told, "Tell us if there's a problem," rather than, "This is what we're doing." And yet, I'm the one who's actually made the plea for help!

Suzie viewed making a BIT report as asking for help with a student. She did *not* view making a report as moving the issue off her plate and onto another's. In this example, this student was still in and attending her class. She explained how "they [BIT] took it, and I know a bit more about this now, but they took it as, a referral, that once it's in their jurisdiction, it's out of mine." This is problematic as Suzie is the person seeing and working with the student on a weekly basis, not members of the BIT.

She explained how this particular situation made her "furious" and how it felt like a "betrayal." She wondered "What the hell did I do this for?" The main issue for Suzie was "now he [the student] knows it's me. He knows that I've referred him." While Suzie made the BIT report in an effort to access help in working with a student, the situation had become untenable. She assumed the student no longer trusted her because she made the report, which necessarily impacted the learning environment.

Suzie also told a story about a class wherein "a young male student . . . took a very strong fancy to a young female student, and started stalking her, basically, all around campus." The situation became tenuous. Suzie explained the students "went out on a date, [but] she didn't like him, and didn't want to go out again, and he started just following her, and arguing with her, an-and eventually yelling at her, and then grabbing her by the arm." The student experiencing this interpersonal violence came to Suzie and was "very, very upset."

Suzie made a BIT report, and upon doing so, she inquired about how best to handle the situation. Recall that both of these students were in her class at the time. She asked "'What am I supposed to do about this?'" She was bereft when she realized "they can't tell me," and went on to say "I understand there's confidentiality, all the rest of that. . . . [but] it's just you [faculty] on the front line." These types of situations further illustrate the tensions faculty experience when navigating these institutional structures and systems.

Harriet explained a situation wherein she made a BIT report upon experiencing stalking by a student. She noted "I used it [BIT] only in the circumstance of this student who was, kind of, stalking me. . . . I am reluctant to do that, because we have no control over how those records are then used." It is interesting to see here, that even in the face of her personal safety being at risk, she was hesitant to make the report.

This was another example of how some faculty viewed the BIT as a punitive body and the BIT report as something that could harm a student's future. Upon probing more about this, Harriet said

> Well, for one thing, they don't [students' records], they're not, they're not erased. They stay there. And we have had circumstances in the past, where [clears throat] there were some slip-ups in the information that the faculty member thought was confidential. [The information] was later shared with the student or was shared with someone else.

Confidentiality breaches such as this one are problematic but not likely widespread. Yet one bad experience can taint perceptions about the integrity of the process.

Harriet explained she "see[s] the BIT reports—and maybe this is my own misunderstanding—really more in terms of disciplinary action, or taking action versus expressing a concern that this student is having." In other words, she saw a BIT report as trigger for institutional disciplinary action—not as a mechanism to express concern or request a student be referred to campus resources.

Phoebe, a full-time instructor within Legal Studies, mentioned making BIT reports only in life-threatening circumstances, as noted below. In this case, it was her life that was being threatened. Here again faculty reluctance to engage in BIT reporting is seen—even in this extreme and precarious example: "[t]he last time I used the BIT was when the—the kid [student] said he was gonna bring a gun in and shoot me. I reported that because I thought that deserved to be reported." To be sure, this was an incident that warranted a BIT report.

Phoebe explained further "I don't like to use them [BIT] because, they say, 'Oh, they're not on their permanent record,' but I know that they can be accessed." She also mentioned other institutions being able to gain access to the BIT records. She said "I know that they can be accessed by other institutions. . . . They tell you that they aren't, but they can be. And they can be accessed if these people want to be police officers or get involved in law enforcement." This is a significant reason why she only makes BIT reports in extreme cases.

Like some of the other faculty in this study, Phoebe mentioned that she does not "use them [BIT] unless it's something [extreme] like that [threat of gun violence]." She typically relied on her ability to work directly with the student of concern rather than enlisting others. She noted "I very rarely file a BIT report. I usually go directly to the student and try to work it out with them."

Justin had so much experience with mental health issues as a social worker, he has never filed a BIT report. He handles the issues on his own. In addition, because he teaches in the evening, he has never referred a student to counseling because "those guys are long gone by the time I even get on campus." With his vast knowledge of the resources available within the community, he can refer students elsewhere.

Again, several faculty noted not being willing to submit a BIT report unless the situation was dire. Christina, who had been at the institution for 13 years, had never made such a report. She explained

> I've never done a BIT report. . . . I would have to have a student that would get violent [before submitting a BIT report]. Or show me that they're, like, on the edge of hurting themselves—or like a complete breakdown. . . . I'm not going to put something like that on a student's record because it follows them. . . . to file a BIT report on a student would be really huge.

Corroborating this, Stephanie made BIT reports as a counselor in the past, but not as a teacher. Her insights provided an interesting dual perspective. She explained "I haven't had to do one as a teacher." However she continued by saying "in situations where, because of my counseling background, situations where I probably, probably would have done a BIT report, other faculty would say, 'Oh no, I, you know, that's not to the level that I would have done.'"

This change in perspective based on position is important. Faculty social-ization and the establishment of norms related to the BIT ought to be further interrogated. Stephanie said straightforwardly: "many faculty wouldn't do [BIT report] one unless it's something really severe."

While this will be discussed more in the next section of the book, processes in place meant to alert institutional personnel about instances of plagiarism or academic dishonesty, threatening or violent on-campus or in-class behaviors, and students in need of support (e.g., mental health, basic needs) should be decoupled. Because the BIT reporting process is viewed as punitive—often both by student and reporters—faculty referral agents view BIT reporting as an undesirable option when it comes to supporting student mental health. They consider it a last resort, not the start of a helping conversation about how to best support the student.

Harriet, who has been at the college for 15 years and is a full-time English instructor with tenure, went on to explain BIT reporting is inextricably con-nected to the academic dishonesty policy:

> Well, actually, the thing that we were looking at with the academic dishonesty policy [is that] within five days of discovering [an instance of academic dishon-esty,] faculty are required to enter a BIT report. Well, first of all, how I handle plagiarism, in my class, or academic dishonesty, is based on my judgment in terms of the severity of it, the repetition of it, the intent. I'm not going to . . . I am not going to submit a BIT report. That is something that I think is within my prerogative, and my responsibility to handle. I don't want that appearing because I think that's highly prejudicial.

Harriet saw managing a plagiarism issue as something she ought to handle on her own, as an extension of her pedagogical practice, which makes sense considering her discipline.

Students may unknowingly plagiarize within an English class because they have not yet learned about acceptable citational practice within academic writing. Many times, students need development, not punishment. The BIT may not be able to provide that development. This is likely another reason why the BIT is viewed as an agent of punishment and record keeping.

Marie also provided evidence that perhaps the BIT be bifurcated. One arm could be dedicated to problematic behavioral issues and the other dedicated to referral to services. The main issue seemed to be that reports meant to be referrals were maintained on a student's permanent record, which would have negative impacts down the line. In 17 years, Marie made just one BIT report. She noted submitting a report

> only if I thought the student was going to act out. A student that was cheat-ing, or something like that, I don't know if I would go to that length. But I

would obviously confront them or whatever, but I wouldn't, it wouldn't, I wouldn't feel, unless they were making me uneasy that I would be writing BIT reports on them.

Joy, an adjunct faculty member who taught within Human Services at the institution for 28 years while working full-time within private practice, had a different perspective on the BIT. It was still very much viewed as a punitive body. For example, she mentioned making a BIT report in response to student plagiarism, which often results in some kind of restorative and/or punitive action by the institution, depending on the details of the incident.

At the same time, and perhaps because of her background, experience, and expertise, Joy reported *knowing what happens* upon submitting a BIT report. Again, this may be because of her proactivity and unique skill set. She said "if I'm directly involved, I would find out what happened. . . . if it's something that involves me, I always know. I've never been in the dark." Because of this participant's background and time spent with the college, she may be better equipped than most faculty to support students with mental health concerns, navigate campus structures, and effectively share campus resources with students.

## SUMMARY

While it may seem that having mechanisms in place to facilitate the referral of students to counseling services and other resources on campus (e.g., disability services, campus food pantry) and the BIT is unquestionably good, faculty have many different perceptions of and orientations to these referral and reporting systems and structures. There were rampant frustrations about the lack of feedback upon referring a student to counseling.

To faculty, feedback loops were seen as left open and unclosed, which caused consternation. Counselors urged faculty to share what they knew about any given referred student but would not (could not) provide information or updates in return. If these communication loops were, in fact, closed, it seemed as though faculty, the referral agents, were never looped back into the communications. This was a source of stress for faculty, especially if referred students were back inside the classroom. Faculty felt ill-equipped to best work with that student while being kept in the dark.

Some faculty did not make referrals to on-campus counselors because they taught at night, and there were no longer any counselors on campus. Some, because of their experience and expertise, referred students directly to community resources best suited to assist. In a sense, this type of referral may be more efficient, especially if there are limits to and restrictions on what a campus-based counselor is able to provide (e.g., three one-hour counseling sessions per term). Faculty also viewed the BIT reporting process as problematic.

At this institution, the BIT was seen as a punitive body by many of the students and faculty. There was a conflation of roles played by the BIT; it seemed to be a catch-all for reporting students' threatening or violent behavior, academic dishonesty, and mental health concerns. There was a sense that making a BIT report equated to placing a dark mark on students' permanent record, which could have negative future impacts on students' ability to be considered for employment, transfer to a four-year institution, and be seen in a positive (or at least neutral) light by whomever may have access to those records at the institution and beyond.

Decoupling these multiple functions of the BIT may help resolve some trepidations among faculty and students. Many faculty consciously decided to side-step the referral and/or BIT reporting process to benefit students. These faculty sought to manage any given issue on their own, which in some cases meant violating institutional policy (e.g., not submitting a BIT report for a student who plagiarized).

This behavior may be viewed as prosocial rule-breaking among faculty;[3] see Martin's quote at the start of this chapter. In other words, these faculty are (sometimes) knowingly bending or breaking rules to benefit students—and student success, by extension. The final section of this book will include recommendations related to helping institutional leaders understand how these referrals are perceived and how they can become more effective.

## NOTES

1. Thomas R. Bailey, Shanna Smith Jaggars, and Davis Jenkins, *Redesigning Americas Community Colleges: A Clearer Path to Student Success* (Cambridge, MA: Harvard University Press, 2015); Harry J. Holzer and Sandy Baum, *Making College Work: Pathways to Success for Disadvantaged Students* (Washington, D.C.: Brookings Institution Press, 2017).

2. Bailey, Smith Jaggars, and Jenkins, *Redesigning America's Community Colleges*; Scott A. Bass, *Administratively Adrift: Overcoming Institutional Barriers for College Student Success* (New York: Cambridge University Press, 2022).

3. Amanda O. Latz, "Leveraging Prosocial Rule Breaking among Community College Adjunct Faculty," Journal of Applied Research in the Community College 29 no. 2 (Fall 2022): 125–134. https://www.montezumapublishing.com/jarcc/issueabstracts/fall2022volume29issue2.

## Chapter 9

# Making It Work

"[A]lways have compassion because a lot of our students are going through hard times."

–Rose

As quoted in chapter 1, Alan Schwitzer and John Vaughn said they "know that professionals from every corner of campus can describe firsthand how students' mental and physical wellness, or lack thereof, can affect their learning and success."[1] These authors also asserted that "being on the lookout for student wellness concerns, approaching students who appear in need, and following through—must be the gold standard."[2]

Most of the faculty involved in this study met that gold standard. They made it work. Working with students who may have mental health issues or challenges was an acknowledged part of their jobs, and they found ways to work with all their students.

As articulated earlier, some of the most innovative, effective, student- and content-centered, artful, and thoughtful pedagogies unfold within the community college sector. This may be a function of necessity, as there is no typical student.

Eve explained this phenomenon well when she shared that her community college students represent "different religions, different ethnicities," and different abilities. Two of her students had American Sign Language interpreters during the term she was interviewed. Her students are "young" and "older," covering a vast spectrum of ages. And speaking of spectrums, she continued that some of her students "are actively engaged" and, at the same time, she had one student who "was sleeping this morning" in her class.

The community college, in many ways, is akin to a one-room schoolhouse. There is potential for so much diversity, and faculty must evolve constantly to meet the needs of their students. Carolyn, for example, derived a strategy for encouraging a student on the autism spectrum to be more participative in class. The student asked her to never call on them unless their hand was raised. They made a deal, and it worked.

Not only did these faculty share some of the strategies they used when working with students regarding mental health, they also provided examples of advice they would give to new faculty at their institution. The advice provided by participants was drawn from their own experiences with students—along with reflection on what had worked and what did not work.

Many faculty provided hypothetical advice to new faculty by concretizing many elements of their own pedagogical ontologies, including knowing students, engaging in care work, deploying affect-conscious pedagogies, and being a student of students. Having the skills and knowledge set necessary to act as a referral agent was also noted.

In terms of advice she would provide a new faculty colleague, Rebecca focused on learning relevant policies and procedures (i.e., knowing what to do), including submitting a Behavioral Intervention Team (BIT) report, and asking for help and support. Time and experience are faithful teachers, as she noted a lot is learned by "osmosis." She cautioned that while it is okay to call students or send them a note if you have a concern, "there is a limit [to what can be done]."

Helen emphasized the importance of talking with students. She mentioned that students may be or feel vulnerable because of some of the things they are experiencing. She encouraged asking students "what they need in that moment." Providing specific options can be helpful as well; sometimes students may not know what they need when in a moment of crisis. Some options may be stepping into the hallway, having a drink of water, sitting down, doing a deep breathing exercise, walking to the counseling center, or calling someone for a ride home.

Sophie also highlighted the importance of knowing students as a faculty member by keeping lines of communication open. Students should feel supported. Knowing the resources surrounding them at the college can foster this feeling. She said:

> I think it's important to have open communication with the students. So, depending on what course you're teaching, get to know your students. In every course, I want to know every student's name. I want to have a personal conversation with them, at least one time. Just to get to know them, you know. "Hey, how are you today? Um, how's this going?" I think those personal connections are really important to student success.

She also advised faculty to let their students know about all the support resources available to them. Make sure students know that "there's a support team here for them."

Trust is an important part of communication. As noted earlier, many community college students have had negative educational experiences and, accordingly, view educational agents as threatening. Jody encouraged new faculty to "try to enlist [students'] trust and showing sincere interest in their wellbeing." She believes "establishing rapport" with students and showing them "you're truly wanting to care" will help students open up and minimize the chances that they might think any "punitive response" might happen if they suggest they are struggling with something and need help.

Christina noted the criticality of paying attention to students, which was emblematic of an affect-conscious approach. She said, "students tend to take on challenges differently, it affects them differently, and you really need to watch your students when you're teaching them, and working them, and see how they're responding."

Christina also said she can sometimes sense anxiety in her students' eyes and body language. When that happens, she says, "you've got to let them know that there's support for them, that there's ways to deal with stress, and they could talk to somebody, whether on campus, or off, outside of campus, or whatever." Faculty can play an important role to encourage students to "find the help" they need, so they can "deal with stress and anxiety" in effective ways, so that "it doesn't overwhelm them."

Students should be constantly reminded of the resources available to them through the college and the community. Joy emphasized that the college and the community need to be linked if students are to access and benefit from available resources. She also mentioned the importance of being proactive by keeping an updated list of resources and contact information in course syllabi and using the institution's learning management system to communicate information and resources.

Because there is no such thing as a typical community college student, Sophie also noted the importance of flexibility. She said, "We have a wide variety of students here. So, one policy doesn't always work. It can't always be, 'Okay, these are my office hours, and that's it.' There has to be some flexibility."

Phoebe encouraged working *with* students to generate solutions to whatever they may be facing that is affecting their success in the course. What may work for one student may not work for all students. Marie expressed similar sentiments. When she hires new adjuncts, she makes sure to tell them to be "flexible." For example, she discourages new adjunct faculty from having a rigid attendance policy or insisting on no make-up exams. "You have to be willing to be flexible," she said.

Harriet cautioned against making assumptions about students. She opined: "I have a feeling I would be amazed at what's really going on in my classroom if I knew everybody's story." She also stated:

I think one thing is to just be aware of your students, and to realize that they will change a lot in the course of this semester, so that, not to jump to any conclusions. . . . Try to listen to what's going on, and, you know, there are some ways. Like, I, lots of times, will talk to students after class and just say, "Could I talk to you for a minute, you know, I thought you seemed upset about this." . . . Be aware that you have to be very careful not to assume that everybody's had the same experience.

Compassion was noted as an important characteristic and default position when working with students. Rose advised to "always give [your students] a chance to explain themselves," and be compassionate. Rose also connected acting with compassion to not making assumptions about students.

Based on her previous teaching experiences, Rose shared, "I never judge a student." She has had students with cancer and with other challenging medical conditions who were juggling a lot of struggles in life. And sometimes those struggles are not health related. She shared the story of one student she almost made the wrong assumptions about:

He sat in the back and he'd nod off in class and . . . almost all classes he'd nod off. And, you know, I could have thought, "Oh, come on. You know, wake up. Pay attention." Turns out he was an EMT who worked all night and then came right to class. . . . So, you know, I tell people don't, you know, don't judge them until you know what the circumstances are.

She advises faculty not to judge, rather "just express your concern." Ask your students if they are okay, for example. Teaching with compassion is key "because you have no idea what's going on in their life."

## SUMMARY

Despite encountering many challenges, these faculty made it work. During the interviews, they shared insights related to how they would advise new faculty on working with students who may be managing mental health concerns, illnesses, or disorders. Without question, these faculty practiced what they preached.

In many ways, the advice they would offer was emblematic of previous chapters in this text about their dispositions and pedagogies, how they view students' assets and obstacles, doing emotional labor, not seeing students with mental health concerns as a monolithic group, and how they navigated institutional structures and systems. The final section of this book is focused on actions community colleges can take—immediately and in the future—to further support their students.

## NOTES

1. Alan M. Schwitzer and John A. Vaughn, "Mental Health, Well-Being, and Learning: Supporting Our Students in Times of Need," *About Campus* 22 no. 20 (May/June 2017): 4–5, https://doi.org/10.1002/abc.21287.

2. Schwitzer and Vaughn, "Mental Health, Well-Being, and Learning," 5.

# PART IV

# The Future

This book is part of a series on the future of community colleges. When considering the most recent data available on the prevalence of mental health concerns among community college students coupled with the current and projected future state of the world and nation, community college student mental health will not soon improve. Therefore, the final two chapters are dedicated to what can be done now and what can be done in the future related to supporting community college students' mental health.

As has been emphasized throughout this text, there are no panaceas for this issue. Ideas put forward in this section are not meant to be prescriptive. They need to be adjusted for context. Work on this issue must be thoughtful, intentional, grounded in data, informed by the literature, and modified over time as contexts change. Chapter 10 is dedicated to the present, or what can be done in the immediate, and chapter 11 is pointed toward the future, or what can be done once those immediate steps are taken.

# Chapter 10

# What Can We Do Now?

"I would love to put my [social work] practicum students over there [in counseling] doing case management and referral and education and all of that. That would be a phenomenal practicum."

–Joy

The purpose of this chapter is to help readers consider where to begin most immediately when it comes to supporting community college student mental health. This is a complex issue and requires thoughtfulness, care, and evidence-based strategies.

## THE IMPORTANCE OF FRAMING

One of the first things that can be done immediately regarding the issue of community college student mental health is to consider the way it is being thought about, conceived of, and mentally framed. Like most issues within higher education and the community college sector specifically, this issue is complex and nuanced.

Work on this topic will necessarily involve messiness, and that should not be ignored. Instead of rejecting that reality, fully embrace the complexity, nuance, and messiness of the issue. For example, and as was presented earlier, not every student with a mental health concern is the same. It is critical to reject monolithic conceptions and concomitant blanket fixes.

There is no silver bullet solution to this issue. In fact, there *is no* concrete solution to this issue. There are only ways to manage it and provide students with as much support as possible. Just like physical health, everyone has mental health, and health fluctuates during the life course for everyone. It is important to embrace this reality rather than turning to fatalism or cynicism.

Complex issues require thoughtful consideration and equally complex pathways forward. And, sometimes, those pathways forward create more and different issues. That is also to be expected and embraced. Thinking about the issue in this way can help manage expectations about what is possible for institutions and institutional agents to do and accomplish.

Relatedly, it is imperative to recognize that students' mental health concerns are a real and profound issue. Its prevalence among students will, unfortunately, increase; its campus presence and impacts will continue to proliferate. See poor mental health as the norm, not the exception.

There are several reasons why mental health issues have worsened significantly over time and will continue to worsen. For example, the COVID-19 global pandemic was and is a ubiquitous challenge, and it has been particularly challenging for those at the margins of society. While COVID-19 affects physical health, it has also taken a toll on our collective societal mental health.

Climate issues are a present concern for many, and these concerns will continue to become more widespread. Rising temperatures, rising water levels, climate-related migration and displacement, and climate-charged conflicts will continue to pose significant challenges moving forward—both in the US and around the globe. Relatedly, wars between and within nations will also continue to mar global and local landscapes. War motivated by land, resources, and political conflicts will be catalyzed by climate change accelerations.

The ongoing unsettling political landscape within the US shows no signs of relenting. The political arena is highly polarized and polarizing. Recent events, such as the insurrection that occurred on January 6, 2021, have laid bare the fragility of the nation's democracy. National, state-level, and local-level politics will likely continue to be imbued with hate, incivility, intimidation, and fear. Widespread individual and systematic racism and xenophobia continue to place myriad burdens on persons with marginalized racial-ethnic identities. The overturning of Roe v. Wade by the US Supreme Court has caused states to scramble and many have been and will continue to be thrusted into crisis as a result.

Ongoing and widening economic stratification among persons in the US will also continue to be a source of consternation. Deeply entrenched wealth gaps, particularly those connected to race and ethnicity, will persist into the future and potentially widen.

Gun violence and mass shootings within the US have become so frequent they are expected as a daily given. That many of these mass shootings have taken place in educational contexts, while others have been orchestrated against marginalized groups, is deeply unsettling.

State-level anti-trans legislation also places undue burdens on the trans community. In 2021, more than 290 anti-LGBTQ+ bills were introduced throughout the states, and 25 became law.

Lastly, social media and its pull will continue proliferating. This is not an inherently bad thing, but social media can have deleterious effects on users' mental health. Social media can be a great way to remain connected to others, but it can also be a source of anxiety. It can be addictive and a source of unhealthy comparisons. Furthermore, it can shape perceptions of reality through intentionally manipulative algorithms.

In summary, community college leaders should expect and embrace mental health concerns among their students. Students are managing a lot right now, and the loads they carry will likely continue to become heavier. Again, we all have physical health, *and* we all have mental health. And that health is not always good. Ups and downs lasting a variety of lengths of time are normal throughout the duration of the life cycle.

## Normalize Trauma and Trauma-Informed Approaches

Another element of this reframing is to normalize students' trauma experience(s). Prior to the COVID-19 global pandemic, it was shown that the overwhelming majority (89%) of community college students had experienced at least one traumatic event within their lifetime and that community college students experience trauma more and more severely than their four-year institution counterparts.[1]

High prevalence and severity of trauma exposure leads to poor outcomes in a variety of domains, including mental health and student success measures, such as GPA. After having experienced a pandemic, it should be assumed that *all* community college students are entering with trauma histories. Most community college personnel likely know this intuitively, but efforts should be made to normalize that reality.

Trauma-informed approaches to working with community college students should be adopted to account for this reality. In fact, community colleges—in both their physical and online iterations—should be transformed into trauma-informed spaces. One way to think about trauma-informed approaches is moving from the question *What is wrong with you?* to *What is happening to you?* The latter question acknowledges that students' trauma is not just in the past; it lives on into and affects the present.[2]

Using grounded theory, Nicholas A. P. Mortaloni et al. built a Trauma-Informed College Model, which includes two key elements: trust at all levels and equity-mindedness.[3] In addition to these two key elements, there are five key themes within the model, each creating the foundation for the subsequent theme:

- First, the institution must assume responsibility for supporting students by using trauma-informed approaches across campus. Buy-in from the board, executive leadership, administrators, and others in leadership positions on campus is vital.
- Second, a coordinated effort to institutionalize trauma-informed approaches must be deliberately executed.
- Third, professional development for faculty and staff is paramount. This includes increasing awareness, skill building, and resource sharing.
- Fourth, individuals must commit to trauma-informed approaches through acting accordingly. This includes using life experience with trauma to foster empathy, being empathic with words and actions, noticing and taking action when a student is struggling, balancing nurture with structure, following through on promises, and referring students to resources.
- Fifth, and finally, universal design is meant to connote the cultural-embeddedness of trauma-informed approaches throughout every aspect of the institution.[4]

Models and guides like this one can help community colleges consider holistic ways to better support their students.

## View Student Mental Health as an Equity Issue

Ignoring equity gaps is no longer an option for community college leaders. Sarah Ketchen Lipson et al. asserted that "[c]ontinued research on the unique mental health needs of community college students is imperative in promoting equity . . . and funding for mental health services on community college campuses is a high priority."[5] Institutional action on this equity issue is necessary.

Recently Estela Mara Bensimon and Yolanda Watson Spiva reframed the term *equity gaps* to *institutional performance gaps*, which moves the focus from students' socio-demographic characteristics to the actions of the institution.[6] This language change reaffirms that the onus for bridging the gaps rests on institutions, not students. While this framing may seem overwhelming to institutional leaders, it should be a comfort. Institutional actions are controllable.

There is a robust literature available on equity-mindedness, equity assessment, and addressing equity gaps.[7] Community college student mental health is most certainly an equity issue—one that can be considered, assessed, and addressed. This is not to say that community colleges, or their leaders by extension, are expected to solve students' mental health issues. However, it is imperative that community colleges take action to remove barriers faced by students and introduce support to students who are managing mental health issues.

As was made evident in the first section of this book, because of the complexity of this issue and the vast diversity of community college students, there are equity issues inside equity issues, making this work arduous. Rest assured it is worth the effort.

When working through equity assessments, disaggregating data based on several variables is key. For example, when looking at student mental health data, disaggregating by race and/or ethnicity could be illuminating. There are deeply rooted negative mental health stigmas within many Asian and Asian American cultures.[8] Examining whether Asian and Asian American students who screened affirmatively for a mental health concern access resources at the same frequency as their peers could help inform practice meant to address that equity gap if one exists.

## COLLECT, DISAGGREGATE, SHARE, AND USE DATA

Data are essential to any effort to support community college student mental health. You must know your students before enacting initiatives, interventions, or policies. It is critical to assess students and responsibly share the data—in the aggregate and in disaggregated forms—across campus widely.

### What to Assess?

There is no shortage of items that could be assessed during data collection efforts. However, students' time is valuable, and survey or assessment fatigue is real. At the start of this process, two major categories of decisions must be made. The first is what information should be gathered from students. The second is which mental health concerns or illnesses should be screened for.

Another consideration is whether anything else ought to also be screened for or assessed such as food or housing insecurity, financial stress, or the use of certain coping mechanisms. The extant literature on this topic can provide guidance. Existing student data is another source of guidance.

Although not an exhaustive list, it may be apt to collect the following information from students when carrying out mental health screenings: race and/or ethnicity, gender, sexual orientation, (academic) program, veteran status, student-athlete status, whether the student has been diagnosed with a mental health concern, whether the student has been to counseling or therapy, and whether the student is taking medication as a mental health treatment.

To be sure, no student should feel forced to share any personal or health information they do not want to share. It should be made abundantly clear to students that they should only share what they feel comfortable sharing. Although data may be incomplete as a result, having this type of information allows for disaggregation, which can show patterns. It can also be used to expose equity gaps.

Another consideration is which mental health concerns ought to be screened for. This may include depression, anxiety, suicide ideation, non-suicidal self-injury, and eating disorders. Relatedly, it may also be helpful to assess student attitudes and behaviors regarding their academic performance, help-seeking, counseling, mental health knowledge, mental health stigma, and knowledge of warning signs or red flags.

## When to Assess?

When to engage in assessment is also an important consideration. Assessment should occur at a time when students are actively engaged in coursework but not during a particularly busy time such as the midterm or the week before a long break. It would not, for example, be advantageous to assess students between terms, during the summer, or on a national holiday. However, consider your institution's academic calendar and plan accordingly. Other assessment initiatives on campus should be considered as well. For example, sending or administering three surveys to the entire student body in one week is not a good idea.

Related to when to assess is how often to assess. Assessing too frequently will harm response rates. Assessing the entire student body more frequently than once per year should be questioned. It may be useful, however, to assess before and after interventions. On only rare occasions would a whole-population intervention be deployed. For example, if a whole-campus marketing and communication campaign was executed to combat negative mental health stigma throughout the academic year, it might make sense to assess at the start and end of that year. Frequency of assessment depends on contexts. Often less is more.

## How to Assess?

There are at least two ways to engage in this sort of assessment. The first is to contract with an outside entity to complete the assessment. The second is to carry out the assessment independently or internally. The first option would be costly, while the second would be complex and require time, resources, and a team of personnel. The second may also require outside assistance.

Organizations that engage in this type of work include the American College Health Association, the Healthy Minds Network, and the Center for

Community College Student Engagement. The following can be administered by an outside entity:

- American College Health Association-National College Health Assessment III (ACHA-NCHA III). This can be costly, and community college students are underrepresented in reference group data. Information on how to participate can be found at the ACHA website (https://www.acha.org/NCHA/Home/NCHA/NCHA_Home.aspx). The fee structure is available online.
- Healthy Minds Study (HMS)—Student Survey. The cost for implementation varies across institutions. Information on how to participate can be found at The Healthy Minds Network website (https://healthymindsnetwork.org/hms/).
- Center for Community College Student Engagement (CCCSE) surveys. Thanks to their Mental Well-Being and Academic Success project, CCCSE is including questions related to student mental health in both their Community College Survey of Student Engagement (CCSSE) and their Survey of Entering Student Engagement (SENSE). More information can be found on their website at https://cccse.org/mental-well-being-project.

Another way to carry out the assessment is to conduct it independent of an outside organization. Community colleges would have to either leverage their institutional research and/or counseling center staff to administer these instruments or work with another entity to do so. For example, a community college could partner with the educational psychology department of a local four-year institution to carry out the study. This work would also make an excellent doctoral dissertation. However, the assessment plan ought to be sustainable.

The following instruments have been used within some of the studies referenced above. Each instrument is focused on depression, anxiety, and post-traumatic stress, respectively. This is not an exhaustive list. There are plenty of available instruments that can screen for a variety of mental health issues, illnesses, and disorders. Many appear free to use, though some instruments may have an associated fee. When in doubt about terms of usage, reach out to the author(s).

- Patient Health Questionnaire (PHQ-9) (see https://www.phqscreeners.com/ for access)[9]
- Generalized Anxiety Disorder Screener (GAD-7) (see https://www.phqscreeners.com/ for access)[10]

- Primary Care Post-Traumatic Stress Disorder Screen (PC-PTSD-5) (see https://www.ptsd.va.gov/professional/assessment/documents/pc-ptsd5 -screen.pdf for access)[11]

The assessment plan should include the collection of quantitative data using a survey. Qualitative data may also provide insights on the topic. Consider using interviews and focus groups. These methods of data collection could include gathering data from students, faculty, and staff. Focus should be placed on understanding trends and issues *and* ways to support students and solve problems. The California Community Colleges created a useful resource (see https://www.cccstudentmentalhealth.org/), which could serve as a template for other state and institutional contexts.

Those who participate in data collection efforts as *researchers* or give their time in service of completing assessments or participating in focus groups as *participants*, for example, should be compensated for their labor. Consider ways to provide that compensation during the planning process. Students' time is valuable, and their financial stress can be significant. Providing compensation is the right thing to do, and it will improve response rates. Strong response rates are critical to building a clear and comprehensive picture of the student body.

Lastly, it could be powerful to involve students in this process. Elyse D'nn Lovell et al.'s work is an excellent example.[12] Students were enrolled in an online abnormal psychology course. They underwent Institutional Review Board (IRB) vetting, received approval for the study, and conducted 14 interviews with family and friends. Online discussion forums were used for data sharing and analysis.

The students' learning was described in the following way: "increased engagement to learn, deepened rather than surface learning, and real-world application applied to their career goals and personal lives."[13] Within this study, students interviewed family and friends. It would likely be feasible to ask students to interview other students in service of these assessment efforts. This should either be embedded into coursework or students should be paid for their labor.

## What to Do with the Data?

First, only collect data you will actually use. Develop an assessment plan with purpose and precision. Again, overburdening your population or sample will have deleterious effects. The purpose of assessment is to understand the student body, which should inform action.

Second, create and close feedback loops related to data collection. Be transparent with all parties regarding data collection, analysis, and use. Work with marketing and communication staff to build campaigns related to the data collection and assessment efforts.

Third, share results widely and responsibly—with students, faculty, staff, the board, community partners, state legislators, and others. Resist framing students using deficit lenses. Share the results in the aggregate and disaggregate the data as appropriate to show patterns, equity gaps, and areas with potential for specific interventions. Remember, data are powerful. Use them to tell the story of your students' mental health.

Fourth, consider what actions will be taken in response to results. In the most immediate, build out 30-, 60-, and 90-day plans. Tools like GANTT charts can be helpful in visualizing and tracking shorter-term planning efforts. Consider who or which units will carry out elements of the plan.

Fifth and finally, determine the ongoing assessment plan. Thinking longer-term, establish one-, three-, five-, and 10-year plans related to these efforts. Furthermore, consider how these data will inform strategic institutional planning. Keep in mind that these plans ought to be made with the understanding that contexts will change over time. The plan should not be so rigid that sensible changes cannot be made. Embrace the inevitability of flexibility and ongoing refinement at the onset of the planning process.

## BRING SOCIAL WORKERS TO CAMPUS

Hiring full-time, on-campus licensed and/or certified social workers to work with students and connect them with resources within the community related to physical and mental health, housing, food, prescriptions, utilities, childcare, Wi-Fi, and legal assistance is a wise investment. Much of the literature on leveraging the skills and expertise of social workers on community college campuses have been driven by increased attention on students' basic needs insecurity, specifically food and housing insecurity. These professionals could also offer students myriad types of support and resources related to mental health.

Yet Marissa O'Neill argued the social work profession has not fully recognized college students as a population in need of their attention.[14] Her study's results suggested social workers need a greater understanding of the challenges community college students face in order to provide support for basic needs security.

O'Neill noted that college students with food insecurity have been overlooked by social workers and wondered "[i]f social workers continue to overlook this population what messages are we sending?"[15] This is a population that requires attention. Furthermore, the *poor college student* trope must be eliminated. It is not a joke. For many, it is a stark reality.

As was noted above, financial issues are a major obstacle for many community college students. Furthermore, many community college students are living in deep poverty, which creates many barriers to basic needs security, which includes access to mental health services. On the other hand, the notion that college students are somehow exempt from receiving what social workers have to offer also needs to be eliminated. Because of O'Neill's study, the community college where the research was conducted collaborated with the county resulting in the local food bank creating a campus-based food pantry.[16]

The food pantry was also a place where the community college students could receive referrals to outside agencies where they were eligible for services. While this model can certainly be efficacious, interns have a regular turnover cycle, which can make sustainability a challenge. Full-time on-campus employees trained and licensed and/or certified within social work would be ideal.

As has been written about previously, many student affairs preparation programs fail to adequately acknowledge and address the community college sector with their curricula.[17] Therefore, program graduates may harbor negative sentiments about the sector, may not be aware of employment opportunities at community colleges, and/or may not be readily prepared to work within the sector.

At the same time, some community colleges have hired graduates of business programs, including bachelor's degree and master's of business administration (MBA) degree holders, to staff their student affairs units, particularly those positions related to admissions and enrollment management. So, graduates of student affairs preparation programs have expertise and experience in student affairs, but that may not transfer to the community college context. And those trained within the field of business may have expertise in sales, project management, and marketing and communication, but not student affairs or the community college sector.

Student affairs staff members may also come from myriad other educational and experiential backgrounds. And while those with preparation in either student affairs administration or business may come into their roles with some knowledge gaps, these gaps can be addressed and developed into strengths on the job.

Adding personnel with social work licenses and/or certifications can enhance the ways the student affairs unit serves and supports students. Bringing these individuals with heterogeneous strengths, expertise, and experiences together through a shared set of values, mission, and purpose through the student affairs division can yield a synergistic environment focused on student success.

In fact, reframing and revisioning student affairs around this central initiative of supporting students' mental health could result in significant shifts in campus culture. The data collected on students' mental health could be a starting point for this work.

## Social Work Practicums on Campus

As articulated by O'Neill, campuses could provide on-campus experiential learning opportunities for aspirant social workers to support community college student mental health.[18] This could involve a partnership with a social work program at a four-year institution. It could also be a peer-to-peer initiative, as was articulated by Joy in the quotation at the start of this chapter.

# CONSIDER TOTAL INSTITUTION VALUES ALIGNMENT

Institutional values are core concepts and beliefs from which the institution operates. These values are grounding. They can be used as a litmus test. For example, asking questions like "Is this investment in line with the values of our institution?" "Are these actions emblematic of our institutional values?" and "Will this initiative further demonstrate our values as an institution?" are important questions to ask when addressing the topic of student mental health.

It is also important to ask whether the values of the institution are the values of sometimes disparate institutional divisions or units such as student affairs, academic affairs, business affairs. Questions should also be asked about how students are viewed, both broadly and from the perspective of different divisions or units. Are they students, burdens, customers, consumers, community members, vehicles for federal and state aid and tuition and fee monies, humans, all the above, or something else entirely? Consider how values and views of students may need to be modified to acknowledge and support students' mental health.

## Build a Care-Centered Campus Culture (and Pay for It)

A care-centered campus is one in which students feel seen, acknowledged, affirmed, validated, loved, safe, and a sense of belonging. But care work is emotional labor, and it is more laborious to care than it is to not care. No longer can we expect community college professionals to engage in copious amounts of emotional labor without compensation. And care cannot be decoupled from emotional labor.

Care and emotional labor are tricky because these concepts are hard to define, codify, and measure. They are often characterized as invisible. But to whom are care and emotional labor invisible? Care and emotional labor are visible and legible to those who give and those who receive. Within the context of this book, the carers and emotional laborers are the faculty. And the students are the receivers.

That said, those to whom this care and emotional labor are invisible and illegible are often those who make decisions about faculty compensation, promotion, tenure (if applicable), and awards. *This* needs to change. Building a care-centered campus culture must include clear articulations of care in institutional values, mission, vision, policies, and procedures. A care-centered campus culture must not simply be a feeling or a vibe. It must be intentionally inscribed into every facet of the institution.

Some examples of this inscription include mandating or incentivizing faculty to spend time with students outside of class through office hours, study groups, or undergraduate research opportunities.[19] This should not be added to an already full faculty schedule. If this is to be added, something else should be taken away such as a course release, reduction of advising load, or reduction of committee service. And if this kind of work is mandated or expected, it should be codified in job descriptions and performance reviews. This codification through policy and procedure can reference institutional values, mission, and vision as substantiation.

Building a care-centered campus culture necessarily takes time. These kinds of changes do not happen overnight. They require intentionality, a team dedicated to the change, and the deployment of a research-vetted institutional change leadership model or process. If this is not presently in reach, smaller-scale initiatives can set bigger changes into motion. For example, providing faculty with material benefits like cash or a course release through awards may be a starting point. Student-generated awards for caring faculty could go a long way in sparking small ripple effects within the institutional culture.

To this end, look to exemplars for guidance but realize context matters. Amarillo College is one such exemplar.[20] The work unfolding there can provide inspiration and templates for other institutional contexts. Know, however, that what works brilliantly at one institution will not work the same way at another. Local context matters greatly. And at the same time, care costs money, and care is costly.

The pursuit of external funding to pay for care may be necessary, at least until compensation for these efforts can be sustainably built into the institutional budget. A starting point may be working with the institution's foundation to raise funds for this important and specific initiative or set of initiatives. Other sources of external monies may include local community foundations, some national foundations, and local, state, and national granting or awarding entities.

The central thesis of Leslie D. Gonzales and David F. Ayers's work is that normalized community college faculty emotional labor is now leveraged by these institutions to make up for the lack of available resources.[21] This is insidious, but in the *do more with less (and less)* environment prevalent within the community college sector from their inception because of inequitable funding, this argument also has merit. Keep this in mind when building a care-centered campus culture and making emotional labor a core responsibility for personnel.

## Consider the Gendered Nature of Care

The gendered nature of care work and emotional labor has long been studied. In general, men do less emotional labor and care work than women and trans and nonbinary individuals. This is evident in the literature on community college student mental health,[22] within this study, and in the broader literature as well.[23] And the weight of this labor can be heavier for women and trans and nonbinary individuals of color because of cultural taxation.

As an example of cultural taxation, if an institution has a large population of Black students but very few Black faculty, those very many Black students may seek support from those very few Black faculty, which can be a lot to manage for those faculty. This is cultural taxation. It is also an equity issue. If the racial-ethnic demography of the faculty mirrored the student body, cultural taxation would be less of a concern. Consider the *many* identities of personnel and students, the gendered nature of care, and the prevalence of cultural taxation in strategic planning efforts.

## TRAIN FACULTY ON THIS TOPIC

Focus on trauma-informed approaches to teaching, advising, and working with students in a general sense. This kind of training is no less important than content-based training or pedagogical training. In fact, consider trainings on approaches that integrate student wellness with pedagogical approaches (e.g., feminist pedagogies) and the ways content may affect students' mental health (e.g., content previews/warnings, clinical experiences). How faculty teach is just as important as what they teach.

While a full articulation of what trauma-informed pedagogies entails is beyond the scope of this book, resources are available. For example, Phyllis Thompson and Janice Carello's edited text on trauma-informed pedagogies includes a community college-focused chapter.[24] The text also contains a robust set of appendices framed as a teaching toolbox.[25]

It is important to encourage faculty to endeavor to understand rather than judge students. As noted above, knowing students is a key to knowing how best to approach supporting their learning. Also, faculty must resist fear when it comes to working with students. To be sure, there may be times when fear is helpful, such as in the event of violence. However, if any given faculty member is fearful of all their students, that is a faculty issue, not a student issue. Seeking to understand students helps alleviate fears rooted in difference.

Faculty should know their roles and the boundaries of their roles. But they should also be encouraged to resist litigious mindsets and tendencies; listening does not require a credential. This is the case for faculty and other institutional personnel as well. Listening to students is a way to get to know them. Taking the time to do so is invaluable insofar as listening to students can inform and improve teaching approaches. It should be emphasized here that feminist, relational, and affect-conscious pedagogies are for *everyone*. These approaches are not relegated to women.

One way to help faculty (and others) develop listening skills is to provide training on some specific helping and microcounseling skills.[26] For example, faculty can be made aware of a set of questions they could use to help a student articulate what they are experiencing or what they need at any given moment. Additional training could include how to understand body language, how to build rapport, how to focus a conversation, and how to respond to students based on the content and tenor of a particular conversation.

While much of the literature on helping and microcounseling is set within the four-year sector and within the context of student affairs, these resources can be invaluable to community college faculty. And they are easily transferable. Certainly, local and individual contexts should be taken into consideration, but learning about and implementing helping and microcounseling skills could be an important part of a community college instructor's took kit when it comes to supporting students' mental health.

Faculty should also be aware of mental health symptomatology and build skills related to supporting students in distress. Mental Health First Aid certification is available and important. This training takes several hours and may have an associated fee, but the certification is something faculty can legitimately place on their resume or curriculum vitae. Browse the web to learn more about offerings in your area. The REDFLAGS model is another important tool that could benefit faculty and should be considered when building training.[27]

Lastly, actively involve faculty in the training. Ask those who are most qualified to lead the training based on their experiences, successes, and/or failures—and pay them for it. Faculty-to-faculty training may be more palatable than training conducted by outsiders. This activity is another item faculty can legitimately place on their resume or curriculum vitae. Consider also asking students to participate as training facilitators or learners.

## ENSURE STUDENTS ARE AWARE OF RESOURCES

If students are to access resources, they must first be aware of them. There are many ways to build students' awareness. At the bare minimum, include mandatory syllabus statements with links to resources. Work with faculty leaders to facilitate this syllabus mandate. Consider ways to build this content into syllabi such that students will be compelled to engage with that content. For example, consider embedding a quick response (QR) code with a link to a Linktree with a curated list of websites containing useful information. If applicable, point students to the on-campus counseling center or social worker(s) as a hub for these resources.

Similarly, this information could be built into a module within the campus learning management system (LMS) and included in all course sites. A task force, which should include personnel from information technology and/or instructional design, could be charged with ensuring updated information is included each term. The inclusion of such a module could be automated, ensuring all students have access to a robust set of up-to-date resources.

Create marketing campaigns that share accurate information about mental health, destigmatize mental health issues, and point students to resources. Consider creating a specific logo for this initiative. Think about high-traffic locations both in the on-campus physical space and online. This may include outdoor signage at the campus entryway, flyers in classrooms, bulletin boards in hallways, digital content in email signatures, and reminders embedded within the campus LMS.

Place this charge into the hands of students and consider building this into the curriculum. Embrace experiential and project-based learning, which could lead to more student buy-in. Leverage interdisciplinary and transdisciplinary teaching opportunities involving psychology, English, communications, business, and arts classes to collaborate on this project. The possibilities are vast.

## RETHINK AND REIMAGINE THE BEHAVIORAL INTERVENTION TEAM (BIT)

State laws that mandate institutions of higher education to create threat assessment teams (i.e., BITs) have proliferated. Models and names vary substantially from campus to campus, and there is a general lack of awareness regarding how these teams function.

According to Gregory T. Eells and Harry S. Rockland-Miller, "[t]he primary consideration in responding to a student's behavior and determining an institutional course of action is understanding that assessment and action must be determined on a case-by-case basis."[28] This cannot be overemphasized and was evident within the study.

Furthermore, three sources of legal standards related to students' information and privacy may be used to guide institutional action. They are (a) The Family Educational Rights to Privacy Act (FERPA), which is federal law; (b) state law and professional guidelines related to sharing students' mental health records; and (c) the Health Insurance Portability and Accountability Act (HIPPA).

Fear and anxiety exist among institutional personnel regarding liability in the event of a student death by suicide or act of violence, and this can often affect how the BIT operates and makes decisions. However, "[w]hen fear of lawsuits becomes paramount there is a risk of defensive practice, which can paradoxically increase risk by detrimentally impacting the decision-making process."[29] A "reasoned and ethical analysis"[30] is the best course of action.

Eells and Rockland-Miller (2011) noted that "the team [BIT] has a responsibility to educate the campus community about its purpose and functioning."[31] Education on how and why to make referrals is also necessary. They also advise "fostering a community culture of caring"[32] through campus-based messaging regarding the team. These points are critical and must be considered. Plus, they flow well from previous recommendations on what can be done right now.

Understand the BIT policies, processes, and communication workflow on campus. It is important to know how the BIT process is perceived by personnel and students, whether it is effective, who it benefits, and why. This could be as simple as asking faculty and student leaders, and it could be as involved as building a whole-campus assessment schema. Determine whether changes or alternatives are necessary based on what is learned.

Outside resources related to BITs and threat assessment exist. The National Association for Behavioral Intervention and Threat Assessment (see https://www.nabita.org/) provides training and certification, resources, and an annual conference. While this organization is not specific to higher education, it includes higher education.

## Decouple BIT Reporting from Other Systems

As was evident throughout the study, faculty had serious concerns about the BIT at their institution. Therefore, it may be necessary to decouple BIT reporting from other systems of referral and notification. Consideration must also be given to who is able to access data related to reporting. What does it mean, for example, if a BIT report exists on a student's *permanent record*? What exactly is a student's permanent record? Who has access to it, and why?

Matters of alleged academic dishonesty, COVID test results reporting, threatening student behavior, counseling center or food pantry outreach, scheduling advising appointments, and disability services should not automatically go through the exact same system, process, or workflow. If using a student success dashboard or management system, it is important to take seriously the confidentiality of student data. Furthermore, some information about students is not relevant to all who may have access. Couple and decouple systems and processes related to student mental health with intentionality and thoughtfulness.

## WORK WITH INSTITUTIONAL LOBBYISTS

Work with both in-house and/or contracted institutional lobbyists to educate local government officials, state legislators, and policy makers about this issue, with an eye on coalition building and public support. Consider a palette of approaches. Consider how to translate data into compelling narratives and presentations. Many of those in positions to pull policy levers know nothing about what contemporary community college student life is like. Change this.

Furthermore, enlist local news media in efforts to bring attention to the issue in terms of the prevalence of student mental health issues and the innovative ways a college is providing support to students who need it. Work with marketing and communications professionals as well as legal counsel to convey messages thoughtfully and responsibly. Again, involve faculty, staff, and students in this messaging.

## WORK WITH FOUNDATION PERSONNEL

Leveraging the institution's foundation to support a care-centered culture was mentioned above but working with the foundation's personnel regarding this issue is vital in a broad sense. Examples include raising funds to provide faculty with Mental Health First Aid certification, bring additional mental health counselors from the community to campus a few times a week, participate in a student health assessment, or purchase an institutional subscription to a mental health app.

Better supporting students requires money. Connect with foundation personnel to generate campaigns to raise monies to support the many initiatives above that may require substantial resources. While community colleges and their personnel are used to unfunded mandates, they are problematic. Consistently doing more with less is not a sustainable model. As mentioned above, conducting assessments and responsibly sharing data can bring awareness and attention to this issue, which can lead to funding sources.

## LEVERAGE TECHNOLOGY WHILE ACKNOWLEDGING ITS LIMITS

Most community college students have smartphones. Mobile health (mHealth) communication is a promising way to deliver mental health services to college students. The literature suggests that (a) mHealth can increase students' awareness of available resources and the dimensions of wellness, (b) mHealth is effective in transmitting information and delivering interventions to students, and (c) students are open to the idea of mHealth and willing to try it out.[33]

Focus on in-house application (app) development and/or purchase institutional subscriptions to extant apps. Think about how mental-health focused resources could be included into extant in-house apps used by students. Many students access and complete coursework through their phones. It may be possible to build mental health resources into the institutional LMS, which could be easily accessible to students through the LMS's app, which is already likely widely used by students.

Consider regional or state-wide multi-institutional subscriptions to lower costs. One-stop shops are best in this case. For example, rather than purchasing subscriptions to four different apps, one each for making an appointment with the counseling center, guided meditation, learning coping skills, and connecting to mental health care providers, subscribe to an app that can do it all.

App affordances may include appointment scheduling, links to resources ranging from local providers to lists of positive coping strategies, guided meditation, and even tele-counseling. While mHealth and mental health apps are useful, they are not a cure-all and should be one part of a holistic support plan for students.

## SUMMARY

The purpose of this chapter was to outline what institutions can do about this issue right away. Recommendations herein were conceived of based on the research on this topic, the study upon which this book is based, and personal experiences. It is vital to continue emphasizing the importance of institutional context. What works at one institution could be a disaster for another.

The contents of this chapter are not meant to be prescriptive; they are meant to be suggestions. Upon engaging the assessment process, much will become apparent regarding next steps—both in the immediate and in the future. The final chapter of this section and the book is centered around what can be done in the future.

# NOTES

1. Samantha L. Anders, Patricia A. Frazier, and Sandra L. Shallcross, "Prevalence and Effects of Life Event Exposure Among Undergraduate and Community College Students," *Journal of Counseling Psychology* 59, no. 3 (2012): 449–457, https://doi .org/10.1037/a0027753.

2. Janice Corello and Phyllis Thompson, "Developing a New Default in Higher Education: We Are Not Alone in This Work," in *Trauma-Informed Pedagogies: A Guide for Responding to Crisis and Inequality in Higher Education,* eds. Phyllis Thompson and Janice Carello (Switzerland: Palgrave Macmillan, 2022), 1–12.

3. Nicholas A. P. Mortaloni et al., "Creating a Trauma-Informed College Model for Improving Student Success," *Community College Journal of Research and Practice* (2022), https://doi.org/10.1080/10668926.2022.2050840.

4. Mortaloni et al. "Creating a Trauma-Informed College Model."

5. Sarah Ketchen Lipson et al., "Mental Health Conditions Among Community College Students: A National Study of Prevalence and Use of Treatment Services," *Psychiatric Services* 72, no. 10 (October 2021): 1132, https://doi.org/10.1176/appi.ps .202000437.

6. Estela Mara Bensimon and Yolanda Watson Spiva, "The End of 'Equity Gaps' in Higher Education?" *Diverse Issues in Higher Education*, August 24, 2022, para 3, https://www.diverseeducation.com/opinion/article/15295980/the-end-of-equity-gaps -in-higher-education.

7. Estela Mara Bensimon and Lindsey Malcom, eds., *Confronting Equity Issues on Campus: Implementing the Equity Scorecard in Theory and Practice* (Sterling, Virginia: Stylus, 2012).

8. Meekyung Han and Helen Pong, "Mental Health Help-Seeking Behaviors Among Asian American Community College Students: The Effects of Stigma, Cultural Barriers, and Acculturation," *Journal of College Student Development* 56, no. 1 (January 2015): 1–14, https://doi.org/10.1353/csd.2015.0001.

9. Kurt Kroenke, Robert L. Spitzer, and Janet B. W. Williams, "The PHQ-9: Validity of a Brief Depression Severity Measure," *Journal of General Internal Medicine* 16, no. 9 (2001): 606–613, https://doi.org/10.1046/j.1525-1497.2001.016009606.x.

10. Robert L. Spitzer, Kurt Kroenke, and Janet B. W. Williams, "A Brief Measure for Assessing Generalized Anxiety Disorder: The GAD-7," *Archives of*

*Internal Medicine* 166, no. 10 (2006): 1092–1097, https://jamanetwork.com/journals/jamainternalmedicine/fullarticle/410326.

11. Annabel Prins et al., *Primary care PTSD screen for DSM-5 (PC-PTSD-5)* [Measurement instrument] (2015), https://www.ptsd.va.gov/professional/assessment/documents/pc-ptsd5-screen.pdf.

12. Elyse D'nn Lovell et al., "Online Community College Student-Researchers Explore Mental Health Stigmas: Deeper Learning Implied," *Community College Journal of Research and Practice* 44, no. 4 (2020): 308–311, https://doi.org/10.1080/10668926.2019.1666065.

13. D'nn Lovell et al., "Online Community College Student Researchers," 311.

14. Marissa O'Neill, "The Effect of Social Support on Community College Students Experiencing Food Insecurity: An Overlooked Population," *Social Work & Social Sciences Review* 20, no. 1 (2019), 63–77, https://doi.org/10.1921/swssr.v20i1.1144.

15. O'Neill, "The Effect of Social Support," 74.

16. O'Neill, "The Effect of Social Support."

17. See Amanda O. Latz et al., "Student Affairs Professionals in the Community College: Critically Examining Preparation Programs From a Social Justice Lens," *Community College Journal of Research and Practice* 41, no. 11 (2017): 733–746, https://doi.org/10.1080/10668926.2016.1222507; Dan W. Royer et al., "Looking Back From the Field: Student Affairs Practitioners' Perceptions of a Graduate-Level Community College Course," *Community College Journal of Research and Practice* 40, no. 3 (2016): 237–241, https://doi.org/10.1080/10668926.2015.1112320; Danny W. Royer et al., "Making Community College Student Affairs Visible in Master's-Level Student Affairs Preparation: A Longitudinal Curricular Analysis," *Community College Journal of Research and Practice* 45, no. 7 (2020): 535–539, http://doi.org/10.1080/10668926.2020.1771627.

18. O'Neill, "The Effect of Social Support."

19. Nancy Hensel, *Undergraduate Research at Community Colleges: Equity, Discovery, and Innovation* (Sterling, VA: Stylus, 2021).

20. See Marcella Bombardieri, "Colleges Are No Match for American Poverty," *The Atlantic*, May 30, 2018, https://www.theatlantic.com/education/archive/2018/05/college-poor-students/560972/; Sarah Goldrick-Rab and Clare Cady, "Supporting Community College Completion with a Culture of Caring: A Case Study of Amarillo College," *Temple University and Wisconsin HOPE Lab*, June 2018, https://tacc.org/sites/default/files/documents/2018-08/wisconsin-hope-lab-case-study-amarillo-college.pdf.

21. Leslie D. Gonzales and David F. Ayers, "The Convergence of Institutional Logics on the Community College Sector and the Normalization of Emotional Labor: A New Theoretical Approach for Considering Community College Faculty Labor Expectations," *The Review of Higher Education* 41 no. 3 (Spring 2018): 455–478, https//doi.org/10.1353/rhe.2018.0015.

22. See Sarah Ketchen Lipson, Amber Talaski, and Nina Cesare, *The Role of Faculty in Student Mental Health* (Lexington, MA: Mary Christie Institute, April 2021),

https://marychristieinstitute.org/wp-content/uploads/2021/04/The-Role-of-Faculty-in -Student-Mental-Health.pdf.

23. See Anne Statham, Laurel Richardson, and Judith A. Cook, *Gender and University Teaching: A Negotiated Difference* (Albany, NY: SUNY Press, 1991).

24. Jeanie Tietjen, "Naming the Urgency: The Importance of Trauma-Informed Practices in Community Colleges," in *Trauma-Informed Pedagogies: A Guide for Responding to Crisis and Inequality in Higher Education,* eds. Phyllis Thompson and Janice Carello (Switzerland: Palgrave Macmillan, 2022), 113–124.

25. Phyllis Thompson and Janice Carello, eds., *Trauma-Informed Pedagogies: A Guide for Responding to Crisis and Inequality in Higher Education* (Switzerland: Palgrave Macmillan, 2022).

26. Monica Galloway Burke et al., eds., *Helping College Students in Distress: A Faculty Guide* (Oxfordshire, England: Routledge, 2021); Monica Galloway Burke et al., *Helping Skills for Working with College Students: Applying Counseling Theory to Student Affairs Practice* (Oxfordshire, England: Routledge, 2016); Amy L. Reynolds, *Helping College Students: Developing Essential Support Skills for Student Affairs Practice* (San Francisco, CA: Jossey-Bass, 2009).

27. Michael T. Kalkbrenner, "Recognizing and Supporting Students with Mental Health Disorders: The REDFLAGS Model," *Journal of Education and Training* 3, no. 1 (February 2016), http://dx.doi.org/10.5296/jet.v3i1.8141.

28. Gregory T. Eells and Harry S. Rockland-Miller, "Assessing and Responding to Disturbed and Disturbing Students: Understanding the Role of Administrative Teams in Institutions of Higher Education," *Journal of College Student Psychotherapy* 25, no. 1 (2011): 9, https://doi.org/10.1080/87568225.2011.532470.

29. Eells and Rockland-Miller, "Assessing and Responding," 11.

30. Eells and Rockland-Miller, "Assessing and Responding," 11.

31. Eells and Rockland-Miller, "Assessing and Responding," 19.

32. Eells and Rockland-Miller, "Assessing and Responding," 19.

33. Kaprea F. Johnson and Michael T. Kalkbrenner, "The Utilization of Technological Innovations to Support College Student Mental Health: Mobile Health Communication," *Journal of Technology in Human Services* 35 no. 4 (2017): 314–339, https:// doi.org/10.1080/15228835.2017.1368428.

*Chapter 11*

# How Might the Future Look?

"[Community college students] want to get an education. For some students, they're the first person in their family to go to college, and that's a big deal. . . . you see the families there [at graduation] and the response, and, you know, they're just really proud."

–Eve

While there is much to do immediately about this issue, longer-term visioning and planning is also essential. We cannot predict the future. Yet we can envision ideal futures and work toward making them reality. At the same time, institutional leaders must be nimble and understand and account for the changing landscapes in which students are living their lives, which affect their mental health.

## TAKE AN ECOLOGICAL VIEW

Students do not exist acontextually. See each student as the center of a complex and layered ecology. Students who are managing mental health concerns may also be managing other kinds of challenges such as accessing affordable childcare, securing housing, and experiencing various forms of oppression based on identities. Taking an ecological view can help illuminate these complexities and contexts.

Urie Bronfenbrenner's ecological model could be a helpful tool for understanding as illustrated by Michael T. Kalkenbrenner, Amber L. Jolley, and Danica G. Hays.[1] According to this model, individuals exist within several nested systems, from smallest to largest: the microsystem, mesosystem, exosystem, and macrosystem. In addition, the total ecosystem exists within a chronosystem; this means it exists through the passage of time.

The chronosystem also accounts for changing contexts. Each level within the ecosystem includes different things, though there can be some overlap between levels.

There are several levels. The microsystem includes those persons and institutions closest to the individual such as the immediate family, friends, faith community members, and schools. The mesosystem includes entities like health and social services and extended peer groups; the mesosystem can also be seen as a "system of microsystems."[2] The exosystem includes elements of mass media and popular culture, bodies of government, and socio-economic status. The macrosystem includes systems and forces that impress upon global realities like colonialism, white supremacy, capitalism, and patriarchy.

Bandages may help and get students through to the next moment, but they do not solve long-term, deeply rooted issues. While keeping in mind what it ought to look like presently, considering it was originally conceived of nearly 50 years ago, Bronfenbrenner's model can be used to gauge where influence can be made and to brainstorm ways to take precise and substantive action.[3]

For example, consider that, because of globalization, something happening in the macrosystem might be directly and profoundly affecting a group of individual students. For example, global supply chain issues may lead to an extended hospital stay if certain medical supplies are not available. Routine car services could be delayed for days and weeks for the same reason. These inconveniences could be catastrophic for community college students and negatively impact their mental health.

Consider what can be done structurally, economically, or at the policy level to alleviate undue strains students may be facing. Use the model to identify toward which point within the ecosystem you will target your intervention(s). Recall that each system is subsumed by the next. The systems are porous and will continue to compress into one another as the world shrinks because of myriad technologies like the internet and ubiquity of smartphones with cameras. For example, the violence and carnage happening locally *and* across the globe can be consumed with ease through social media.

## ENGAGE IN STRATEGIC PLANNING

Build a long-term, temporally based strategic plan focused on this issue. Alternatively, build this issue into the next strategic planning cycle. Consider goals relative to student mental health. Ongoing assessment can help establish benchmarks from which specific, measurable, attainable, realistic, and timely (SMART) goals can be derived, tracked, and met. Rather than thinking in terms of days and months, consider years and decades.

Doing this work well involves time, a team, committee, or task force dedicated to the work, and a vetted process. There are resources available and examples to review. The Jed Foundation and the Education Development Center, Inc. created a *Guide to Campus Mental Health Planning*, which includes three sections: building momentum and infrastructure, engaging in a strategic planning process, and strategies for promoting mental health and preventing suicide.[4]

The Jed Foundation also offers partnerships through Jed Campus.[5] Jed Campus helps institutions with program and policy development meant to support student mental health through either a four-year or 18-month partnership. During the four-year partnership, year one includes assessment and strategic planning. Years two and three are dedicated to implementation and support. Finally, year four is about evaluation and sustainability.

Vanderbilt University's Strategic Plan for Vanderbilt's Mental Health and Well-Being can be accessed online.[6] This plan was created by a committee and set into motion by the Chancellor. This strategic plan is not just focused on students; it is focused on the entire campus community. Recommendations within the Plan were separated into sections dedicated to the whole campus community, students, and faculty and staff. There are also dedicated recommendations sections meant to address campus culture and how to position the institution as a national leader on research in this area.

A focus on mental health can also be folded into the broader campus strategic planning cycle. For example, many community college strategic plans include sections dedicated to one or more of the following: student experience, student success, and equity. This is precisely where an emphasis on mental health could be added.

Yet what works best for one institution may not work at all for another. Context should inform how to frame this important element of the strategic plan. Lorain County Community College couched mental health within efforts to expand wrap-around services.[7] This was framed as a means to increase completion and academic success among students. On the other hand, Grand Valley Community College situated supporting students' mental health needs as part of their equity strategic goal.[8]

## INTEGRATE ACADEMIC AND STUDENT AFFAIRS

Dismantle silos and question hierarchies. Review the espoused organizational charts and workflows, then see what is happening in service of students. Consider whether there is any formal overlap between academic and student affairs. View faculty as student affairs practitioners; view student affairs practitioners as educators. Though their parts in the process may vary, at their core, many of these professionals envision similar outcomes for their students. All campus personnel should be involved in the work of supporting student mental health.

Post critical questions about relationships and partnerships such as: "How are our units working with one another?" "What is working well, and what needs improvement?" "In what ways does disability services work with tutoring services?" and "Are faculty aware of the food pantry's hours of operation?" Look for ways to further integrate what can be very disparate divisions and units. Reward collaborations and partnerships in service of supporting student mental health and its correlates (e.g., financial stress, housing insecurity) with internal grant monies to the extent possible.

## INVOLVE THE BOARD

Upon creating student assessment cycles, create a communication plan related to those data that involves the Board. Just as college personnel need to know their students, so, too, does the Board. And Boards will require data to support decision-making at the executive level. Board members could be a valuable resource in addressing and redressing this critical issue.

## BUILD UP SUPPORT FOR PERSONNEL

Secondary trauma and compassion fatigue are real. Employee burnout is also real. Its effects are deleterious to students. Faculty working conditions must be taken seriously. As alluded to by Gary Rhoades, faculty working conditions are student learning conditions.[9] Building a care-centered culture should not stop with student-focused care. That is where it should start, not where it should end.

Support for personnel must include adequate compensation and access to resources, a supportive work environment, and acknowledgment of emotional labor. Be mindful of inequities related to who is doing emotional labor. Understand and address cultural taxation. Ask who among your professional community is doing the most emotional labor. Consider assessing to understand, and then pay these individuals accordingly—or at least acknowledge the work.

## MOVE INTO THE MISSION

Community colleges are notorious for having an exaggerated sense of a reasonable mission—or set of missions. While we have long thought of missions as being related to transfer preparation, career and technical education, workforce development, developmental education, community education, and so on, what about the cultivation of student wellness, of a comfortable and safe environment where learning can flourish, of a student body that understands the primacy of physical and mental health? Consider whether institutional mission needs to be addressed as part of the process of building support systems for students' mental health.

## ENGAGE WITH THE COMMUNITY

Community colleges are powerful educational, social, cultural, political, and economic institutions. Use that power—and influential capital—for good. Upon taking an ecological view of the contexts in which students exist, imagine what can be done to ameliorate (some of) the unjust systems, policies, and/or in place that may be contributing to students' mental health concerns. Then act.

Encourage personnel to become active within the community—and beyond. This means membership on not-for-profit organizations' boards, which could facilitate collaboration and team-based problem solving. It also means heightened civic engagement at all levels—local, state, regional, national, and international.

Data are powerful. Who our students are—including their lived realities, their many assets, and the obstacles they are made to overcome—should not be a secret. As appropriate, share information about the student body with the community. This could be a powerful way to mobilize and leverage support for student support initiatives that will benefit both students and communities. This could also be a vital step within an ongoing capital campaign. Map community assets related to this issue and forge mutually beneficial relationships that target this issue.

This is not an issue to be addressed by a task force or an ad hoc committee. Working on this issue effectively requires all. This work must be institutionalized. This is another opportunity to take an ecological perspective. It is also another opportunity to consider framing. It is important to decouple mental health concerns and illness and danger, fear, and violence. Again, all of us have mental health. This is not a topic to shy away from or ignore altogether.

Involving everyone goes beyond personnel at the institution. Understand what is happening in local high schools as it relates to mental health. Understand what is happening within the local community as it relates to mental health. Create relationships and work groups that connect high school counselors, community college faculty and student affairs professionals, and mental health leaders and practitioners within the community. Connect with the National Alliance on Mental Illness (NAMI) at the local, state, and national levels. It is also important to understand what is happening at receiving transfer institutions as it relates to mental health.

It is of utmost importance to educate and train campus police and/or campus security personnel on this issue. Center data, trauma-informed approaches, and cultural competency. Consider topics such as (racial) profiling, stereotype threat, and (racial) battle fatigue.

## SUMMARY

The state of community college students' mental health is not good, both in absolute and in comparative terms, and it is likely to worsen over time. The purpose of this chapter was to outline ideas and recommendations for shaping the future of how community colleges support their students' mental health.

Again, the suggestions contained within this chapter are meant to be suggestive, not prescriptive. This work, like anything worthwhile, is difficult. Doing this work, however, could change campuses and change lives. The hope is that this chapter, the one before it, and this entire text become a part of the good work that will continue unfolding with the nation's community colleges in service of the students who depend on them for education, to be sure, but also liberation.

## NOTES

1. Urie Bronfenbrenner, "Toward an Experimental Ecology of Human Development," *American Psychologist*, 32, no. 7 (1977): 513–531, https://doi.org/10.1037/0003-066X.32.7.513; Michael T. Kalkbrenner, Amber L. Jolley, and Danica G. Hays, "Faculty Views on College Student Mental Health: Implications for Retention and Student Success," *Journal of College Student Retention: Research, Theory & Practice* 23, no. 3 (November 2021): 636–658, https://www.doi.org/10.1177/1521025119867639.

2. Bronfenbrenner, "Toward an Experimental Ecology," 515.

3. Bronfenbrenner, "Toward an Experimental Ecology."

4. The Jed Foundation and Education Development Center, Inc., *A Guide to Campus Mental Health Action Planning,* 2011, https://sprc.org/sites/default/files/resource-program/CampusMHAP_Web%20final.pdf.

5. The Jed Foundation (website), *Get Started with JED Campus,* 2021, https://jedfoundation.org/jed-campus/.

6. Vanderbilt Chancellor's Strategic Planning Committee, *Strategic Plan for Vanderbilt's Mental Health and Wellbeing,* December 2017, https://www.vanderbilt.edu/wp-content/uploads/sites/3/2021/08/Strategic-Plan-for-Vanderbilt-Mental-Health-2018.pdf.

7. Lorain County Community College (website), *Vision 2025,* https://www.lorainccc.edu/about/vision-2025/.

8. Grand Rapids Community College (website), *Strategic Plan,* June 2022, https://www.grcc.edu/faculty-staff/instructional-support-institutional-planning/strategic-planning/strategic-plan-202225.

9. Gary Rhoades, "Taking College Teachers' Working Conditions Seriously: Adjunct Faculty and Negotiating a Labor-Based Conception of Quality," *The Journal of Higher Education* 91, no. 3 (2020): 327–352, https://doi.org/10.1080/00221546.2019.1664196.

# Appendix A

## *Methodological Overview*

This study was originally conceptualized using a constructivist grounded theory methodology.[1] However, upon building this book, it became apparent that a different approach to the data analysis was necessary to create a more accessible text, one useful for practitioners. Therefore, during the writing process, I engaged in reflexive thematic analysis to organize and present the data.[2]

As mentioned in the body of the text, I conducted 22 interviews with community college faculty about their perceptions of and experiences with their students' mental health. These interviews took place in January and February of 2017. All interviews took place in person and in a location convenient to the participant. The shortest interview was 35 minutes and the longest was 86 minutes. Following each interview or day of interviewing, I created detailed notes about my experiences and emerging interpretations. See Appendix B for the interview protocol used.

Each interview was transcribed by Rev (see https://www.rev.com/). The transcription turnaround was usually less than 24 hours. Interview transcripts were analyzed in several phases. I reviewed my notes, then listened to the audio recording while correcting or *cleaning* each transcript housed within a Word document. Transcripts were also rendered confidential through supplanting names and locations with pseudonyms or generic replacements (e.g., [city]).

Analysis began with the note making process and continued into a formalized and systematic process wherein I listened again to the audio while thematically coding the data transcript by transcript. A separate document was built where I listed codes and supporting evidence for each code from each of the transcripts, where applicable. This included my own interpretations of the data along with verbatim interview transcripts. I then organized the codes into broader categories, which became themes and subthemes. These themes and subthemes were embedded, in part, as headers and subheaders throughout the text.

Even in writing a book based on this study, its totality is not fully conveyed. While I have presented elements of this study at national conferences, the work has not been published elsewhere (e.g., in the form of a journal article). The data were so important that a complete telling was necessary. The complete telling is this book. However, it remains incomplete. I could have written forever on this topic, as its unfurlings are ongoing. What is contained in this book, however, is everything I could muster up in service of the community college leaders—and others—who need it most.

## NOTES

1. Kathy Charmaz, *Constructing Grounded Theory,* 2nd ed. (Thousand Oaks, CA: Sage, 2014).

2. Virginia Braun and Victoria Clarke, *Thematic Analysis: A Practical Guide* (Thousand Oaks, CA: Sage, 2022).

# Appendix B

## *Interview Script and Protocol*

**Script** [to be read to participants]: *Thank you for agreeing to participate in this interview with me today. Before we get started, I would like to take a moment to go over the informed consent document.*

[go over informed consent document; answer any questions; ask participants to complete and sign two copies of the informed consent document; keep one signed copy; provide the second copy to the participant]

*I appreciate your completion of the informed consent document. We are now ready to start the interview. I will turn on my audio recording device now. Let us begin.*

1. Tell me about your professional journey to becoming a community college faculty member.
2. Tell me about your faculty position at [community college].
   a. What courses do you teach? In what format are those courses offered? Approximately how many students populate those courses?
   b. What does your teaching load look like? How many courses do you teach?
   c. What, if any, other responsibilities do you have in this position outside of teaching?
   d. Are you employed full-time at [community college]? If no, do you have other employment?
3. What do you like most about teaching within the community college environment in general?
   a. What do you like most about teaching at [community college]?
4. What is most challenging about teaching within the community college environment in general?
   a. What is most challenging about teaching at [community college]?

5. What is your favorite teaching story?
6. What are your students like?
   a. What is a "typical" [community college] student like (e.g., demographics, academic performance)?
   b. Do the courses you teach attract a specific "type" of student? If yes, please explain.
   c. Over the course of the time you've worked at [community college], have you noticed any trends in terms of the students you typically see in your classes or otherwise work with as component of your faculty position?
7. What are the most significant barriers your students face in pursuing their educational goals?
8. What are the most significant strengths they possess in pursuing their educational goals?
9. How prevalent do you believe mental health issues are among your students?
   a. Are certain student subgroups more likely to have mental health issues? Please explain.
   b. If you believed a student was experiencing mental health issues, how would you know? Are there specific "flags" or symptoms you look for? If yes, what are they?
   c. If you believed a student was experiencing mental health issues, what would you do?
   d. How do mental health issues present themselves inside a classroom?
   e. Could you share a specific story about a time when a student's mental health issue became apparent inside a classroom?
10. Of the students dealing with mental health issues that you have known, tell me about the nature and severity of those issues.
   a. What are some of the most common mental health issues or diagnoses students seem to face (e.g., anxiety, depression, bipolar disorder)?
   b. Could you share a specific story about working with a student with mental health issues?
11. How are students with mental health concerns supported at [community college]?
   a. What else could [community college] do to support students with mental health issues?
12. How aware are students regarding the mental health resources available to them—resources both on and off campus?
13. How safe do you think students feel when they are on campus?
   a. What leads you to believe this?
   b. Can you give a specific example of what you mean?

    c. Are certain on-campus spaces safer than others? Why do you think that is the case?

14. How safe do you feel when you are on campus?

    a. What makes you feel safe or unsafe?

15. If you were going to talk with a brand new [community college] faculty member about how to best support students with mental health issues as a faculty member, what would you say?

    a. Do you engage in any ongoing professional development related to students' mental health?

*At this time, I would like to transition into to questions meant to gather basic demographic information.*

16. How long have you been employed as a faculty member at [community college]?

17. What is your highest degree?

18. How do you self-identify in terms of gender and race?

19. What is your age?

20. Thank you for all of your responses. We are nearly finished. Before we formally conclude, however, is there anything else you would like to share with me or any response upon which you would like to elaborate?

*Our interview is now concluded. Thank you so much for meeting with me today. I really appreciate your participation.*

# About the Author

**Amanda O. Latz**, EdD, is associate professor of Higher Education and Community College Leadership at Ball State University (BSU), located in Muncie, Indiana. In addition to her faculty role, she also serves as director of the Student Affairs Administration in Higher Education (SAAHE) Master of Arts program and director of the graduate certificate in Community College Leadership at BSU. Prior to working at Ball State University, she worked in collegiate athletics, student-athlete support, and within a research center. She also has undergraduate teaching experience, most recently as an adjunct instructor at Ivy Tech Community College. Her research agenda is comprised of two main areas: the lived experiences of students and faculty within the community college and the use of visual methodologies and methods within higher education research. She is an expert on the photovoice methodology. In terms of scholarship, she is an author of two previous books and 40 journal articles, with several other works in the publication pipeline. She is an active member of the Association for the Study of Higher Education, and she serves as a board member for the Council for the Study of Community Colleges. Recently, she was invited to serve on the editorial board for *The Journal of Higher Education*.